ENDOMETRIOSIS

ENDOMETRIOSIS

ENDOMETRIOSIS

THE NAME OF THE PAIN
AND HOW TO REPRESS IT

LEONARD WEATHER JR., RPH, MD, FAPCR

ENDOMETRIOSIS

The Name of the Pain and How to Repress it

Copyright © 2023 by Leonard Weather Jr., RPh, MD, FAPCR

1st Edition.

All rights reserved. No part of this publication may be reproduced, distributed, or transmitted in any form or by any means, including photocopying, recording, or other electronic or mechanical methods, without the prior written permission of the publisher, except in the case of brief quotations embodied in critical reviews and certain other noncommercial uses permitted by copyright law.

Book design by Arshad

Tikur Press, Inc.
drweather-endo@att.net

Tikur Press, Inc
2120 Bert Kouns Loop
Shreveport, LA 71118

ISBN: 978-0-9705748-0-0

Printed in the United States of America

DEDICATION

To all the women who have suffered in silence with the pain and challenges of endometriosis, you are brave and resilient warriors who have fought through the agony of infertility, endured the frustration of misdiagnosis, and battled the stigma surrounding women's health.

ACKNOWLEDGEMENT

This book is the result of much more than just my efforts. I would like to express my sincere appreciation to the countless individuals who have contributed to its creation. It has been made possible only through their efforts. I would also like to thank those who have helped me throughout my career, which is a significant component of making this book a reality. From my phenomenal experience with gynecological, infertility and endometriosis training at the Johns Hopkins University Hospital, where I learned from giants such as Drs. Howard and Georgina Jones, who were the first to perform IVF in the US, to my collaboration with Dr. Donald Chatman, the first to adequately report endometriosis in Black women via his seminal paper, "Endometriosis in the Black Woman." Additionally, I have gained valuable knowledge from giving presentations on endometriosis and other gynecological disorders while attending the National Medical Association (NMA) Ob/Gyn Section meetings, NMA regional and annual meetings, and from my many years of involvement with the American Association of Gynecologic Laparoscopist (AAGL), the Endometriosis Association, and more recently, the Academy of Physicians in Clinical Research.

I would like to offer many thanks and praises to Dr. Joseph Hicks, Dr. Cynthia Montgomery, Valerie Davis, and others for their assistance, thoughtful contributions, and detailed editing, which have made this book as readable and clear as possible. I would like to

iv | ACKNOWELDGEMENTS

thank my patients who have allowed me the honor and opportunity to diagnose and treat their endometriosis, which has caused them pain and/or infertility.

Finally, I express my gratitude to the readers of this book, whose interest in endometriosis has the potential to promote awareness, knowledge, understanding, and compassion to assist those who live with this challenging condition, "endometriosis, the name of the pain without a name."

FOREWORD

The 21st Century opened with a new respect for women's health and healthcare needs. Women were now asking for more information about their health and conditions that might affect them. Print and visual media were now publishing articles about conditions that affect women's wellbeing. Women no longer just accepted what they were told about their bodies, but demanded more information and to participate themselves in determining how their bodily changes or health threats would be approached by the medical community. They want more information about prevention and preservation of good health across the lifespan. They also now expect to play a role in deciding how their conditions should be diagnosed or treated, and to know more about alternatives to traditional forms of therapy or if newer techniques or interventions exist. Women want to know if surgical interventions are necessary or if alternatives to surgery exist.

As efforts to address research on conditions that affect women's health have become better appreciated, women no longer want to be excluded from clinical research or trials, and now ask what has research shown and what are the most recent scientific advances about conditions of concern. They want to be included as volunteers in approved investigative research studies. Scientific journals increased their publication of studies of women and even new scientific publications came into existence to provide the increased attention to, and demand for, outcomes of increasing research and other studies about women's reproductive, mental, and other conditions that affect both men and women but may affect women differently. These changes reflect the modern women's health movement. Women have long been recognized as the major decision maker for health and medical care for their families, but now are demanding, and receiving, evidence-based information to better execute their roles in that decision making.

Despite advances in attention to women's health and expanding that concept beyond the reproductive system, inclusive of total bodily issues across the lifespan, there are still some very prevalent health concerns for which the answers have not been defined. Specifically, the affliction of endometriosis has remained as an often little understood but major cause of pelvic pain, sometimes infertility, and other related symptoms and ill effects on women. And the related issues of uterine leiomyomas (fibroids) and adenomyosis continue to cause morbidity for women. So that is why this publication by Dr. Leonard Weather, Jr. is a valuable contribution for women as well as their health care providers.

As Dr. Weather notes in this timely and much needed book, '...endometriosis is not a one size fits all chronic condition.' He further states that 'endometriosis has a profound impact on the quality of life' for women worldwide and can be the cause of symptoms that may range from annoying to debilitating. There are many examples of young or even mature premenopausal women suffering from endometriosis which affects their ability to study, complete their education or maintain their occupational demands.

And, with the recognition that women should be able to contribute to decisions about their treatment options, it becomes imperative to provide a clear, concise, and comprehensive guide to what is known about endometriosis and other conditions that may complicate a diagnosis of endometriosis such as uterine fibroids and adenomyosis. Dr. Weather had done that in this book. He has provided definitions, scientific information about what is known and what needs further exploration, alternative for treatments and related psychosocial, mental, and societal factors.

This is no small matter, as Dr. Weather has reminded us that current data estimate that more than 4 million reproductive-age women in the United States have been diagnosed with endometriosis, and there are likely many more who have not been diagnosed. Seeking better informed and state of the art medical approaches can and will bring relief from the often disabling effects of endometriosis on women and their ability to lead pain free lives with preservation of their fertility.

As Dr. Weather states in this publication, 'Clearly the time has come to minimize delays in endometriosis diagnosis and treatment, which would benefit women worldwide.' His personal dedication to remedy the need for comprehensive and science-based information on endometriosis for the benefit of women and their physicians has resulted in this laudable compilation of what is known and should be known about this condition that will be of great value for all of us.

VIVIAN W. PINN, M.D., FCAP, FASCP

Founding Director (Retired), Office of
Research on Women's Health, National
Institutes of Health

CONTENTS

Dedication	i
Acknowledgement	iii
Foreword	v

SECTION I: DEFINITION AND CAUSE

I.	Introduction	3
II.	Theories on the Cause of Endometriosis	11
III.	Environmental Toxins and Endometriosis	19
IV.	Symptoms	33
V.	Pain and other symptoms of Endometriosis	35
VI.	Infertility and Endometriosis	41

SECTION III: SPECIAL INTEREST

VII.	Fibroid Tumors and Endometriosis	49
VIII.	Adenomyosis and Endometriosis	61
IX.	Cancer and Endometriosis	69
X.	Race and Endometriosis	79
XI.	Unnecessary Hysterectomies	85

SECTION IV: DIAGNOSIS AND TREATMENT

XII.	How Endometriosis is Diagnosed	99
XIII.	How Endometriosis is Treated	109
XIV.	Alternative Ways to Repress Endometriosis	121
XV.	Adolescents and Endometriosis	135

ix | CONTENTS

XVI.	Distant Endometriosis	143
XVII.	Clinical Trials	151
XVIII.	Case Histories of Endometriosis	163
XIX.	Endometriosis Awareness	171
XX.	The Future	175
XXI.	The Epilogue	183

APPENDIX

Glossary	187
Resources	229
Symptoms Tracker	233
References	235
Index	272

SECTION I

DEFINITION AND CAUSE

CHAPTER I
INTRODUCTION

Introduction

Endometriosis is a perplexing and debilitating disease that is often misunderstood and missdiagnosed. Throughout my years of practice. I have noticed that most patients with endometriosis, regardless of race or origin, have one common experience: they have suffered from excruciating pain without a proper diagnosis for a long period of time. This is consistent with the well-known delay of 4-11 years from the first onset of symptoms to surgical diagnosis.[1] According to the Endometriosis Association, the average patient sees five physicians before receiving a proper diagnosis.[2] This delay in diagnosis only adds to the patient's pain and frustration. Many people in their lives, including physicians, health professionals, partners and friends, often dismiss their pain as exaggerated or "all in their head." This is unfortunately compounded by the patient having undergone numerous treatment modalities and surgeries without relief, and without a proper diagnosis. They feel increasingly disappointed and struggle to maintain a normal work and family life. They are in despair, having lost hope that they will ever feel well again.[1]

4 | INTRODUCTION

I'm writing this book out of the enormous concern for women who have endometriosis. It is written for their families, friends, relatives, associates, and health professionals to help them understand what is known about this disturbing disease. I hope to dispel some of the myths surrounding endometriosis and to help these women realize they are not alone. Lastly, I wish to offer them hope by embracing knowledge and quality information in order to achieve peace, better health, and joy.

Population-based data suggest that more than 4 million reproductive-age women have been diagnosed with endometriosis in the United States. As daunting as this number is. It's only telling part of the story, as an estimated 6 of 10 endometriosis cases are undiagnosed. Thus, more than 6.5 million American women may experience repercussions of endometriosis without the benefit of understanding the cause of their symptoms or appropriate management.[3]

When discussing the patient's experience with endometriosis, pain and infertility are usually of greatest concern. These are two of the most common symptoms of the disease, but its impact is even greater. Women with endometriosis suffer from a reduced quality of life, an increased incidence of depression, adverse effects on intimate relationships, limitations in daily activities, reduced social activity, loss of productivity and income, a higher risk of chronic disease, and significant direct and indirect healthcare costs. Furthermore, emerging data suggests that endometriosis is linked to a higher risk of obstetric and neonatal complications.[4]

Endometriosis is estimated to affect 10% of reproductive-age women worldwide, which is approximately 190 million women based on the World Bank's population estimates for 2017. However, the true prevalence of endometriosis is uncertain because a definitive diagnosis requires surgical visualization. Estimates vary widely among different population samples and diagnostic approaches. The prevalence ranges from 2% to 11% among women hospitalized for pelvic pain. Among symptomatic adolescents, the prevalence of endometriosis ranges from 49% for those with chronic pelvic pain to 75% for those with pain that is unresponsive to medical treatment.

Currently, knowledge of population distributions, disease manifestations, and risk factors is limited to data for women in whom endometriosis has been successfully diagnosed. The number and characteristics of undiagnosed cases are unknown. In the future, with more definitive epidemiological and clinical data, perhaps obtained through non-invasive diagnostics, we may learn that everything currently believed about endometriosis, which is biased towards factors associated with access to care, represents only a part of the story.[3,5]

Definition

Endometriosis is a puzzling estrogen dependent disease affecting women in their reproductive years. The name comes from the word endometrium, which is the tissue that lines the inside of the uterus which builds up and sheds each month in the menstrual cycle. However, unlike the lining of the uterus, endometrial tissue displaced outside of the uterus doesn't have a way of leaving the body. The results are internal bleeding, degeneration of the blood and tissue which sheds from the growth, and inflammation of the surrounding areas resulting in the formation of scar tissue.

6 | INTRODUCTION

The displaced endometrial tissue forms lesions, implants, growths, nodules, or cysts of varying sizes. These cysts are known as endometriomas or "chocolate cysts." The implants, growths, and nodules are usually brown, black, or blue in color, but they can also be red, white, tan, or clear and non-cancerous. They are primarily located outside the endometrial cavity. In recent decades, an increased frequency of malignancy in connection with endometriosis has been recognized.[6,7]

Description

Endometriosis lesions can be associated with adhesions. Adhesions are bands of scar tissue that can be comparable to a sprawling spider web. Adhesions can cause organs and tissues in the pelvis to stick together, distort the normal anatomy and prevent normal body functions. Notably altering ovum pickup by the fallopian tubes leading to infertility. These adhesions, lesions, implants, and growths can cause debilitating pain and a host of other problems. The most common locations of the displaced endometrial tissue are in the pelvis - involving the ovaries, the fallopian tubes, the ligaments supporting the uterus, and the area between the vagina and the rectum. They can also attach to the outer surface of and the lining of the pelvic cavity. Sometimes the growths are found outside of the pelvis. They have been found in abdominal surgery scars, notably on the intestines, in the rectum or the bladder, vagina, cervix, and the vulva. Endometrial growths have also been found outside of the abdominal cavity in the eyes, lungs, arms, thighs, and other locations. These are rare and uncommon distant locations.[7]

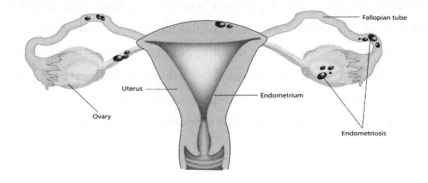

Figure 1. Pelvic Endometriosis

History

Although the claim has been made that there are early descriptions of what today we call endometriosis and adenomyosis in theses presented in Europe in the late 17th and during the 18th centuries; the first description of the condition initially named 'adenomyoma' is that provided in 1860 by the German pathologist Dr. Carl von Rokitansky. Rokitansky was the first to microscopically discover endometriosis in 1860 when he found endometrial glands in the myometrium. It was not until 1921 that this condition was recognized to be of endometriotic origin. The first systematic description of what is today known as adenomyosis was the work of Dr. Thomas Stephen Cullen. He at the turn of the 19th century, fully researched the 'mucosal invasion' already observed by a number of investigators in several parts of the lower abdominal cavity.

8 | INTRODUCTION

It should be clear that there is a close kinship between endometriosis and adenomyosis of the uterus and a frequent clinical association. In adenomyosis the endometrium invades the uterine musculature whereas endometriosis is found at other sites in the pelvis. Both processes show the common property of being misplaced endometrium.[6,8] Cullen clearly identified the epithelial tissue invasion as being made of 'uterine mucosa' and defined the mechanism through which the mucosa invades the underlying tissue. Cullen's observation was made in 1925, this was two years before the term endometriosis was coined by Sampson.

Historically, one of the most consequential tools that has revolutionized the diagnosis and treatment of endometriosis, is laparoscopy. Before laparoscopy became available, endometriosis was often diagnosed through exploratory laparotomy, which involves a large incision in the abdomen. Laparoscopy is a minimally invasive surgical procedure that is typically performed as an outpatient and requires general anesthesia. The use of a laparoscope, which is an attached camera and video monitor, allows for a panoramic view of the pelvis. The abdominal cavity is entered through a single small incision made at the umbilicus (navel), and in some cases, an additional suprapubic incision may be needed for better visualization. The introduction of laparoscopy in gynecology took place in the late 1940s and saw significant improvements over time. In 1967, Dr. Kurt Semm reformed the procedure by enhancing the optical system and the light source and by creating an automatic control of gas insufflations into the abdomen. In 1972, Dr. Henry Clarke patented, published, and recorded a laparoscopic procedure.[9,10,11] Technical advancements in laparoscopy resulted in new knowledge about endometriosis and expanded the use of endoscopic surgery in gynecology.

By the 1970s, leading gynecologists in Europe and the US had concluded that laparoscopy was the preferred tool for diagnosing, staging, and treating endometriosis and other disorders.[6] This was a remarkable achievement that greatly improved the care and treatment of patients with endometriosis.

CHAPTER II
THEORIES ON THE CAUSE OF ENDOMETRIOSIS

What is the cause of endometriosis?

Endometriosis is a complex disease that affects some women from the onset of their first period (menarche) through menopause, regardless of race, ethnic origin, or social status. In fact, it is a global disease, and its exact origin is thought to be multifactorial, as various factors contribute to its development. Several theories have been proposed to explain the origin of endometriosis, some of which will be discussed.[1,2] The following are some of the theories to explain the origin of endometriosis.

Stem Cell Theory

The stem cell theory proposes that the cells responsible for re-establishing the endometrial lining during woman's menstrual cycle may play a role in the development of endometriosis. The spread of these stem cells to unusual regions during the menstrual cycle can lead to the alteration of endometrial cells and cause endometriosis.

Sampson's Theory of Retrograde Menstruation

One of the oldest theories explaining the cause of endometriosis dates back to 1922. Sampson's theory proposes that some of the menstrual blood containing endometrial cells flows backward through the fallopian tubes and into the pelvic cavity. This can occur with or without menstrual blood passing from the vagina during menstruation. It is called retrograde flow. The endometrial cells that flow backwards out of the fallopian tubes implant and bleed. This blood can lead to the formation of scar tissue and further spreading of endometriosis lesions in the pelvic cavity.[3]

Mulleriosis and Embryonic Origin Theory

The theory of mulleriosis proposes that the cause of endometriosis lies in developmental abnormalities in the female reproductive system. The theory proposes that endometriosis occurs due to abnormal changes or movement of any component of the Mullerian duct system. The Mullerian duct system is an area or passage in the growing embryo that develops into the fallopian tubes, uterus, vagina and cervix. [1]

Genetics

There is increasing evidence that genetic factors predispose some women to development of endometriosis. Researchers believe that interactions between multiple different genes, may be responsible for the evolution of the disease. Studies have shown that the risk of developing endometriosis is higher in women who have a close relative who has the condition. Older studies have shown that women with a first-degree relative (mother, sister or child) who has endometriosis have a 7-to-10-fold higher risk of having endometriosis themselves. More recent studies demonstrated that approximately 7% of first-degree relatives of patients with endometriosis also have the disease. [2] A family history of endometriosis has been shown to increase the risk of earlier age of symptom onset, along with similar symptoms, more severe symptoms, and infertility. Researchers are still trying to understand the mechanisms involved in inheritance and the role of genes. It is believed that multiple genetic factors may play a role. A 2019 review of the literature included several studies that focused on the identification of genetic variations related to endometriosis. There were approximately 30 genes associated with the disease in this study. [4, 5, 6]

Environmental

The fact that only some women have endometriosis, implies that there is increased susceptibility to development of disease among certain women. Individual susceptibility is not only influenced by genetic background; but also, by the interaction of genes with environmental factors. Environmental factors may influence cell function by affecting the genome through epigenetic modifications. [7,8] Epigenetic modifications are stable alterations in how a gene makes a protein. The gene sequence; however, is not modified. Studies have shown variations in the epigenetic patterns of genes that play a role in the hormonal, immunologic and inflammatory status of cells in endometriosis. A recent study showed that dietary exposure to dioxin (2,3,7,8-tetrachlorodibenzo-p-dioxin; TCDD) and dioxin-like compounds (DLCs) (*e.g.*, polychlorinated biphenyls [PCBs]) are associated with an increased incidence of endometriosis.[9] Dioxin is a toxic chemical byproduct that occurs in places of uncontrolled

14 | THEORIES ON THE CAUSE OF ENDOMETRIOSIS

burning and recycling of fuels and electronics. Researchers think that dioxin could lead to epigenetic alterations in the DNA and increase the risk of endometriosis. The major route of human exposure to dioxin and dioxin like products is through diet.[10] In fact, more than 90% of typical human exposure is estimated by the Environmental Protection Agency (EPA), to be through the intake of animal fats, mainly meat, dairy products, fish and shellfish.

Other proposed theories

- **Uterine Peristalsis:** Uterine peristalsis, the rhythmic contraction and relaxation of tissue muscle is one of the fundamental functions of the non-pregnant uterus. Contractions of the uterus allow for proper menstruation and are involved in early reproductive processes, such as sperm transportation and egg implantation. Dysfunctional uterine peristalsis may play a part in the development of endometriosis, particularly through the process of retrograde menstruation.

- **Metaplasia:** Overall, the metaplasia theory suggests that the transformation of peritoneal tissue into endometrial tissue is a complex process that involves both hormonal and immunological factors.

- **Hormones:** Researchers have proposed that hormones play a role in the development of endometriosis. Estrogen and progesterone have been a subject of much debate amongst endocrinologists in all sorts of endometriosis theories. More research is needed to fully capture the exact role of estrogen and progesterone in the development of endometriosis.

- **Lymphatic System:** The lymphatic system is part of the circulatory system and is responsible for carrying and removing fluids from the body's tissues. This fluid can contain a variety of essential life components, including red blood cells, white blood cells, and plasma. Many have proposed that this system plays a role in transporting endometrial cells to other parts of the body. This explains how endometriosis can spread throughout the body implanting far away from the uterus. The lymphatic system also serves as a connection for endometriosis involvement with the immune system.

- **Immune System:** The immune system is responsible for protecting the body from disease. In endometriosis, the affected areas become excessively red and swollen. An inflammatory response typically occurs when the body is fighting an infectious disease, the immune system's role in endometriosis progression has become a subject of much interest. Researchers suspect that an issue in the immune system, may make the body ill-equipped to recognize and destroy endometrial tissue growing outside of the uterus.

- **Oxidative Stress:** Free radicals are highly reactive molecules of oxygen. Typically, the body will manage these molecules with antioxidants. Although some free radicals can be beneficial for the body, an excessive amount can be harmful. The elevation of free radicals in the peritoneum (lining of the abdomen) and lack of antioxidants, is suspected to be one of the links in the chain of events that cause endometriosis.

- **Apoptosis:** Apoptosis (the normal degeneration and death of cells) occurs when the body signals out dysfunctional cells which could be harmful and destroys them. This is a highly regulated mechanism and is key in the body's maintenance of preventing disease. In fact, the malfunction in the mechanisms regulating apoptosis is a common cause of cancer. When the body cannot rid itself of harmful and damaging cells, these cells grow, spread and cause tumors and cancer. Endometriosis cells have the capacity to avoid apoptosis. The role this plays in the development of the disease is unknown; however, is currently under investigation. [1,11]

Table 1: Role of the different theories in the development of endometriosis.[12,13]

Theory	Mechanism
Retrograde menstruation	Flow of endometrial content into pelvis, allowing implantation of endometrial lesions outside of the uterus in the pelvic and abdominal cavities
Metaplasia	Transformation of peritoneal tissue/cells into endometrial tissue through hormonal and/or immunological factors
Hormones	Estrogen-driven proliferation of endometrial lesions. Resistance to progesterone-mediated control of endometrial proliferation
Oxidative stress and inflammation	Recruitment of immune cells and their production of cytokines that promote endometrial growth

Theory	Mechanism
Immune dysfunction	Prevention of eliminating menstrual debris and promotion of implantation and growth of endometrial lesions
Apoptosis suppression	Promoting survival of endometrial cells and downregulation of apoptotic pathways
Genetic	Alteration of cellular function that increases attachment of endometrial cells and evasion of these cells from immune clearance
Stem cells	Initiation of endometriotic deposits by undifferentiated cells with natural ability to regenerate
Lymphatic System	Transports endometrial cells to other parts of the body
Uterine Peristalsis	Dysfunctional uterine peristalsis (contraction and relaxation), may play a role in the development of endometriosis

Without question the cause of endometriosis has been studied extensively; however, no single theory is sufficient to explain the development of the disease. It has been suggested that peritoneal endometriosis, chocolate cyst of the ovary and nodules of deeply infiltrating endometriosis are three different disease entities. Each entity is thought to have a different pathogenesis (origination and development). This concept means that diverse pathological conditions underlie endometriosis. It is thought to be a series of syndromes that develop through different mechanisms. In this regard, it's important for research related to determining the specific cause of endometriosis to move forward.[14,15] This will be extremely helpful in the diagnosis and treatment of this disorder.

CHAPTER III

ENVIRONMENTAL TOXINS AND ENDOMETRIOSIS

"Just a word about the word environment': it doesn't just refer to forests, lakes and oceans. It includes our cities, backyards, homes, and bodies. From the air we breathe to the clothes we wear and the furniture we sit on, all are part of our environment. Our bodies reflect the state of the environment around us, and our health is intertwined with the health of our world. When the planet and its environment are diseased with toxic chemicals, our individual bodies can become sick from these chemicals. Therefore, the exact cause of endometriosis cannot be solely explained by genetics, as environmental factors may also be involved. When we use harmful cosmetic products, such as hair dyes, eat contaminated or processed food, or live in houses near plants that emit toxic chemicals, we pollute our most important commodity, our bodies. Fundamentally, we require clean air, water, and food to keep ourselves and our families healthy.[1]

The Mossville, Louisiana Story

The Mossville story is an explicit example of how environmental toxins destroyed an entire town, along with many of the people who lived there. *Mossville was an early settlement of free blacks since 1790. It is in Southwest Louisiana.[2] After the 1940s Mossville became surrounded by industrial plants, which spewed toxic emissions which contaminated the groundwater. Thus, making it "the most polluted corner of the most polluted region in the USA." It is part of an area known as "Cancer Alley."* This area extends **85 miles along the banks of the Mississippi River between Baton Rouge and New Orleans.[3]** The "alley," has a concentration of plastic plants, oil refineries and petrochemical facilities, that together make it one of the most toxic areas in the nation.

In 2014, Mossville was replete with 14 noxious industrial facilities. During the same year SASOL (an integrated energy and chemical company based in Sandton, South Africa), proposed to build the largest chemical plant of its kind in the Western Hemisphere in Mossville. These noxious facilities created what is now known as "the *Louisiana's Chemical Ghost Town Mossville,*" which would all but wipe Mossville off the map. This is due to the harmful effects of the chemicals on the town and its inhabitants. What happened to this town was not initially obvious to its inhabitants, it was like a slow burn. The pernicious chemicals were pervasive, air, soil, water, groundwater, buildings, and structures; causing illnesses such as cancer to those who lived there. We all need to know and be aware of *what's in our neighborhood,* lest the same could happen to us.[4,5,6]

A better understanding of the environmental toxin's impact in Mossville are concerns expressed by *Mossville resident D.F.* *"When I was growing up in the 1950s, we didn't have all this sickness before the industrial facilities came to Mossville. Now, it's so common to know people who frequently go to the doctor for all kinds of health problems. It's scary to find that so many of my relatives and neighbors, are suffering from cancers, endometriosis and asthma. I'm talking about teenage girls with endometriosis and young children who have asthma attacks all the time. I am concerned about the future for my family and my community."*[7]

Women's Hair Products

A recent study highlighted the issue with hair products used by women of color and children. These products contain multiple chemicals associated with endocrine disruption and asthma. The prevalence of parabens and diethyl phthalate (DEP), which is commonly used to help make fragrances last longer, demonstrated higher levels of these compounds in biomonitoring samples taken from Black women when compared with White women. These results indicate the need for more information about the contribution of adverse consumer products to exposure disparities. This is necessary to find out the types, extent of exposure and harm; to design ways to reduce them. A precautionary approach would reduce the use of endocrine disrupting chemicals in personal care products. Furthermore, the labeling of these products should be improved. This would allow women to select products consistent with their values.[8, 9]

Uterine Fibroids

When we embrace endometriosis in the context of reproductive health for women, uterine fibroids are a concern. This concern will be elaborated on in the chapter on fibroid tumors and endometriosis. Aside from the concerns, a study published in the American Journal of Epidemiology, determined that the use of hair relaxers is linked to uterine fibroids in Black women and girls. It is estimated to affect 80% of Black women over their lifetime. The study found two to three times higher rates of fibroids among Black women, when compared to White women. Chemical exposure through scalp lesions and burns caused by relaxers are linked with high fibroid tumor rates. The main ingredients found in relaxers, lye (sodium hydroxide) and no-lye (calcium hydroxide) formulae are linked to scalp lesions and burns. Women who use lye relaxers have a higher risk of scalp lesions or burns. This increases dermal absorption of chemicals directly into their bodies from the scalp. [9]

Reproductive Development

Girls who reported using chemical hair oils and hair perms were 1.4 times more likely to experience early puberty. This was after adjusting for race, ethnicity and year of birth. Other studies have linked early puberty to hair detangler use by Black girls. In one of the studies, African American girls as young as two years old were affected. They began showing signs of puberty after using products containing animal placenta, which are commonly found in many detanglers and conditioners. This information, along with the proliferation of chemicals in hair and beauty products, as well as the possible impacts of untested; unregulated chemicals on Black women's reproductive health, is alarming. African Americans women may be at greater risk today, but it's likely that others may catch up or be in the same position in the future. We need to acknowledge, act on, and redress the problems related to these chemicals posthaste.[9]

Table 2: Beauty Product Exposures [10]

Product Use	Chemical Exposures	Potential Adverse Outcomes
Skin-lightening creams	Mercury	Mercury poisoning, neurotoxicity, kidney damage
Hair relaxers and other hair products	Parabens and estrogenic chemicals from placenta tissue	Uterine fibroid tumors, premature puberty and endocrine disruption
Vaginal douches and other feminine care products	Phthalates and talc powder	Ovarian cancer and endocrine disruption

One needs to ask the question regarding endometriosis. Is there something in our environment, e.g., food, air, hair and cosmetic products, home furniture or water that triggers or causes endometriosis?

Environmental exposure

This is an area in which we need a great deal of research. Research results could offer promising clues about the disease. Studies in rhesus monkeys have shown that environmental pollutants can increase the risk of endometriosis and cancers. In one 1992 study, researchers found that 79 percent of monkeys that were exposed to the environmental pollutant dioxin, developed endometriosis, while those who were not exposed to dioxin had very little or no disease. There was a direct correlation, with the more dioxin exposure in the individual monkey, the greater the endometriosis incidence and severity. Other studies have shown that dioxins and other pollutants can also cause harm indirectly, by disrupting hormone function, which can contribute to endometriosis. [11]

Unfortunately, we do not completely understand the scientific relationship between lifestyle, environment, and endometriosis. There is a profound need for more research in this regard. An important question is, "how can we reduce exposure to environmental pollutants, which may contribute to the disease?"

Mitigation of Environmental Exposure

Several recommendations are presented below which may also be applicable or extended for cancer prevention.

Lower Pesticide, Antibiotic, and Hormone Exposure

Carrying the "USDA Organic," label means that foods must pass strict standards in terms of growth, production, and distribution. The use of pesticides, herbicides, fungicides, genetically modified organisms (GMOs), hormones, and antibiotics are restricted. In lieu of harmful pest control agents, and fertilizers only those that are approved for organic agriculture can carry the label. Non-organic farming uses synthetic chemicals. USDA Organic foods must be completely free of GMOs.

Science has shown us that these organic standards reduce the chemicals in your body, particularly those from pesticides and antibiotics. A comprehensive analysis published in the journal *Environmental Health,* in 2017 concluded that consumers of organic food have significantly lower exposure to pesticides than those eating conventionally grown food. The significance of pesticide contact is evident in the associated increased risk for diseases such as Parkinson's disease, type 2 diabetes, certain types of cancers such as non-Hodgkin lymphoma and childhood leukemia, as well as lymphoma, and cognitive deficits resulting from maternal pesticide exposure during pregnancy or early childhood exposure. [12]

Avoid Contaminated Fish

Found in fatty, oily fish, omega-3 fatty acids can help your heart in several ways. Just a couple of 4-ounce servings of seafood with omega-3 fatty acids each week can lower your chances of heart disease by 36%. Omega-3s might make you less likely to have a stroke and Alzheimer's disease. [13]However, there are some risks associated with eating certain fish on a regular basis. Those high in contaminants such as mercury, polychlorinated biphenyls (PCBs) and industrial waste find their way into lake, and ocean water through the fish who live there and into our household. The Environmental Protection Agency (EPA) and Food and Drug Agency (FDA) have issued combined guidelines. For women of childbearing age, pregnant and breast-feeding women, and children. They advise these groups to avoid fish

26 | ENVIRONMENTAL TOXINS AND ENDOMETRIOSIS

with higher levels of mercury contamination. Fish with high mercury levels include shark, swordfish, king mackerel and tilefish. Alaskan salmon, Artic char, cod, herring, mackerel, mahi-mahi, perch, rainbow trout, sardines, striped bass, tuna, and wild Alaskan pollock have great nutrition and safety profiles. They're eco-friendly responsibly caught or farmed and not overfished. [14]Avoid contaminated fish and be mindful of the fact that *dioxins are concentrated in the dark stripe of the fish.* Check, your state's website for an advisory before eating fresh caught fish particularly predator fish, like bass or scavengers like catfish.

Stop or Limit Plastic Bottle Use

Recent studies show bottled water contain excessive levels of microplastics. These small pieces of plastic debris can be less than five millimeters in size. According to research conducted by Orb Media, 93% of the 11 bottled water brands sampled, all showed traces of microplastics. Their research also showed bottled water contained about 50% more microplastics than tap water. Most bottled water is sold in plastic #1, also known as polyethylene terephthalate (PET). Other studies shows that PET may be an endocrine disruptor, altering our hormonal systems. Although this type of plastic is BPA free, phthalates in bottles can still seep into your water Especially when exposed to high temperatures or stored for an extended period, some companies, such as Poland Spring, use plastic #7 for their 3-gallon water bottles. This type of plastic contains BPA, which has been banned in countries around the world, including the European Union and China, due to its toxicity. BPA exposure is linked to multiple health effects, such as fertility issues, altered brain development, cancer, and heart complications.[15]

Filter Your Water

Filtered water is free from harmful chemicals and other water contaminants. A reverse osmosis system can help remove 99% of the contaminants found in tap water. These include metals such as arsenic, lead, copper, iron, cadmium, and hexavalent chromium. Along with industrial and pharmaceutical byproducts such as pesticides or hormones. In addition, chlorine and chloramine, perfluorooctane sulfonate (PFOS) and perfluorooctanoic acid (PFOA), sediments and particulates. Arsenic is a harmful carcinogenic substance present in unfiltered water; dangerous levels have been known to cause diseases. Aluminum is also often present in unfiltered or poorly filtered water. Though water softener can aid in its removal, traces can remain. Increased consumption can cause liver diseases, hyperactivity, and skin problems. Water filters remove these harmful substances, thus significantly reducing your chances of developing various types of cancer and other diseases related to toxic overload in the body. [16] Thus it's important to filter your water to make sure that the PCBs, lead, mercury, and chlorine are removed.

House Plants May Make Your Home Healthier

House plants may help to make your home healthier via phytoremediation. According to the Encyclopedia of Ecology, phytoremediation is a process; by which air, water and soil are cleansed by plants eliminating some of the pollutants. It's also true that this process can eliminate some dust. Choosing plants that purify the air through their roots and surrounding soil may improve the overall health of your home and yourself. Many plants that are available or used for phytoremediation including snake plants, weeping figs, garden mum, dracaena, aloe vera, peace lily, bamboo palm and spider plant.[17,18] However, spider plants (Chlorophytum comosum) are among the most common and easy-to-mount indoor plants capable of purifying indoor air. They absorb carbon monoxide, formaldehyde, xylene, and many other hazardous gases. These plants are non-toxic and safe for pets and children.[19, 20, 21]

Other aids

No Shoes Inside the House Policy

Removing shoes prior to entering the house decreases the possible transmission of disease-carrying bacteria, along with pesticides, herbicide and other toxins that can be harbored in and tracked from the soles of shoes. Pesticides, herbicides, and other toxins are associated with health risks from minor skin or eye irritation to cancer. [22]

Switch to Chlorine-free Tampons and Sanitary Napkins

In the past few years, scientists and health professionals have voiced growing concerns; relevant to the potential risks of using tampons and other personal hygiene products such as diapers. Increasing evidence suggests some of these products contain trace levels of toxins; that, over time, could pose a significant health risk to those who use them. These toxins include dioxins and phthalates, both classed as endocrine disruptors. Hence the reason why these products are coming under increased scrutiny. New research is now linking the presence of dioxin and phthalates in these products back to the original production process. Dioxin is in the chlorine used to bleach the material and phthalates are added to the plastic compounds in these materials during their production.

If we are to work towards a future in which personal hygiene products are completely safe for human use; society must demand action on three fronts. First, to demand that manufacturers disclose every ingredient in their products. This should be made mandatory on the product packaging. Second, to only accept 100% chlorine-free products. Third, to eliminate use of non-biodegradable plastics from these products. These three steps should give the level of assurances needed to deliver genuine change. [23]

Thus, it's important to switch to chlorine-free paper products, including tampons and sanitary napkins, if possible. Also substitute cloth products for bleached paper products use cloth towels instead of paper towels and unbleached coffee filters.

Use Green Household Cleaners

Standard cleaning products can be bad for health, as they release toxic chemicals into the environment and waterways and can by provoke allergic reactions. Making the switch to natural cleaning products can improve the air quality in one's home, create a safer environment and avoid putting you and your family at risk of long-term health problems. [24] Consider making your own natural cleaning products from simple household ingredients such as baking soda, white vinegar, lemon, olive oil, soap, nuts, or castile soap. [25] Additionally, use green household cleaners or natural ones such as vinegar and baking soda.

HEPA Filters Can Improve Air Quality in Your Home

Air pollution comes from more than automobile exhaust or industrial smoke. Dust mites, mold spores, pollen, and pet dander in the air inside the home can cause problems. If you or your family has allergies or asthma; the use of HEPA filters can trap these pollutants and may help, bring relief.

HEPA stands for *High-Efficiency Particulate Air* and is a type of mechanical air filter. It works by forcing air through a fine mesh that traps harmful particles such as pollen, pet dander, dust mites, and tobacco smoke.

You can find HEPA filters in most air purifiers. These are small, portable units that may work for a single room. Some vacuum cleaners have HEPA filters that trap more dust from their exhaust. These HEPA-equipped vacuums disperse less pollution, along with fewer microscopic dust mites back into the room, while vacuuming which avoids inhalation of toxic chemicals.

Using a HEPA filter in the home can remove most airborne particles that might make allergies worse. However, the particles suspended in air are not the only ones in the home. There are far more in your rugs, bedding, and drapes, and resting on countertops and tabletops. Keeping these areas clean is important, it's also important, when possible, to get rid of the source of allergens and irritants. For example, the only effective way to keep tobacco smoke out of your home is to not smoke or allow others to smoke in your home.

The HEPA filters can be part of a plan to remove irritating and potentially toxic particles from the home. Other parts of that strategy could be to:

- Vacuum frequently.
- Replace carpets with wood, tile, or vinyl flooring.
- Change bedding frequently and wash sheets in hot water.
- Replace draperies and curtains with roll up shades.
- Use high-efficiency furnace filters.[26, 27]
- Get a vacuum with a HEPA filter.

Distinctly, the exact cause of endometriosis is not known, however, there are numerous factors, ranging from genetic to immunological, that may play a causative or facilitating role in endometriosis. The role of the environment is also an emerging factor with growing implications for public health. It is now clear that chemicals in our environment can affect reproduction and reproductive hormones, which can be related to disorders such endometriosis and fibroids.

Implicitly, it is important to better understand the mechanism of action of these environmental pollutants, not only on reproductive health but also on overall individual health. Prevention strategies should include education and setting exposure limits; as well as reducing pollution and improving the use of our natural resources.[28]

Take Away

- It's imperative that we not only know what's in our home and neighborhood. We should also know what's in our food, drink and what we place in our bodies.
- Eat organic as often as possible. Foods that have been grown without toxic chemical are healthier. *The labels will tell the story, make sure to read them.*
- Consider growing organically as many fruits and vegetables as you can for consumption.

SECTION II

SYMPTOMS

CHAPTER IV
PAIN AND OTHER SYMPTOMS OF ENDOMETRIOSIS

Pain

Most women who have endometriosis, surprisingly do not have significant symptoms. However, the most common symptom for women who have endometriosis is pelvic pain. The pathophysiologic mechanisms are not well understood and many women with endometriosis may not have this complaint.[1] The pain is most often cyclic but may also be chronic in nature. The pain usually commences just before menses and continues throughout the duration of menstrual flow and sometimes after. The cyclic lower abdominal pain may favor one side (right or left) or may be in the middle. Intuitively, every woman's symptoms are different. More often than not, the pain and other symptoms tend to get worse as time goes on, unless appropriate treatment is rendered, dysmenorrhea and deep dyspareunia (painful intercourse with deep penetration) are the most common pain complaints with 80% and 30% prevalence, respectively.[1] Painful urination, painful defecation during menses, and intermenstrual pelvic pain are less common, and may be associated with bladder or bowel endometriosis lesions. The pain may also be

36 | PAIN AND OTHER SYMPTOMS OF ENDOMETRIOSIS

noted to occur in musculoskeletal regions, in the flank, low back, or thighs. [2,3] The exact cause of the pain is difficult to ascertain. It is thought to be due to the distinctiveness of the disease process. Actively bleeding lesions can cause discomfort. Pain may also be produced by the production of inflammatory mediators (which act on blood vessels and/or cells to promote an inflammatory response) and neurologic stimulation. It is likely that different types of lesions cause pain through differing pathways. [1]

Infertility

The next most common symptom of endometriosis is infertility. Women with moderate to severe endometriosis, especially those where the ovaries and fallopian tubes are affected by adhesive disease, generally have decreased fertility rates. It is believed. This may occur due to the mechanical obstruction between the ovaries and fallopian tubes, which leads to the failure of gamete transport into the tubal ampulla.[4,5] Many women with moderate to severe endometriosis have undergone surgery for their condition. This can result in decreased amounts of functional ovarian tissue, contributing to their decreased fertility. Interestingly, even women with minimal or mild endometriosis may have decreased fertility compared to those without the condition. The exact cause of this subfertility is still controversial, with some studies indicating that even minimal stage endometriosis is associated with decreased fecundity, while other studies report no effect on fertility and pregnancy outcome.[6] The monthly fecundity rate for normal couples is 15-20%, while the monthly fecundity rate for women with untreated endometriosis and infertility is 2-10%. In addition to the anatomical causes of infertility mentioned previously, there are two other major theories that may explain the decreased monthly fecundity rates seen in women with endometriosis: 1) inflammation and 2) a locally altered hormonal profile. The altered cellular immunity leads to an increase in the number of inflammatory mediators. These activated macrophages create a locally hostile environment that may negatively impact various aspects of reproduction, including sperm function, oocytes, tubes, endometrium and implantation.[7,8,9]

Table 3: Symptoms Associated with Endometriosis [4,9]

Chronic fatigue	Leg pain (one or both) *
Constipation	Lower abdominal pain*
Cyclic lung problems (pneumothorax)	Cyclic Low back pain*
Cyclic shoulder or neck pain	Nausea or vomiting*
Diarrhea* (with menses)	Painful defecation (dyschezia)
Dysmenorrhea *	Painful intercourse (dyspareunia)*
Infertility*	Pain with periods*
Intermenstrual pelvic pain/Non-menstrual pelvic pain *	Pain with urination
Irregular and /or heavy menstrual bleeding*	Pelvic pain*
Joint pain	Cyclic scar swelling and pain

*More common symptoms

Other Symptoms and Associations

Other symptoms of endometriosis can include abnormal menstrual bleeding, diarrhea, intermenstrual pelvic pain, constipation, and chronic fatigue. Symptoms of extra-pelvic endometriosis, such as cyclical shoulder pain and cyclical spontaneous pneumothorax. This may also include cyclical cough, or nodules that enlarge during menses.[10, 11] (Table 3), Furthermore, patients with endometriosis may have elevated rates of autoimmune diseases, such as hypothyroidism, interstitial cystitis, and rheumatoid arthritis, lupus erythematosus, Sjögren's syndrome, and multiple sclerosis. [4,7,11] Reports of allergies, asthma, chronic fatigue syndrome, and fibromyalgia are also more common in women with endometriosis than in women in the general US population. [8]

Table 4: Autoimmune Diseases Associated with Endometriosis [9,10,11]

Autoimmune thyroiditis	Interstitial cystitis
Celiac disease	Lupus erythematosus
Fibromyalgia	Multiple sclerosis
Hypothyroidism	Rheumatoid arthritis
Inflammatory bowel syndrome (Crohn's disease and ulcerative colitis)	Sjögren's syndrome

Endometriosis is not a one size fits all chronic condition and every woman's symptom may be different. It's apparent there are a host of symptoms related to endometriosis, some are annoying and others disturbing and even debilitating. [9,10,11] The opportunity and decision for treatment or treatment type should be the woman's call, along with consultation and guidance with her gynecologist.

There is little correlation between the extent of endometrial lesions and severity or duration of symptoms. Some individuals with visibly large lesions have mild symptoms, while others with few lesions have severe symptoms. Symptoms often improve after menopause, however, in some cases painful symptoms can persist. [12, 13, 14] Chronic pains, may be caused by pain centers in the brain becoming hyper-responsive over time (central sensitization). This can occur at any point throughout the life course of endometriosis. Central sensitization can be seen in treated, insufficiently treated, and untreated endometriosis. This may persist even when endometriosis lesions are no longer visible. [15,16,]

Take Away

You may find it useful to record your symptoms using a symptom diary or tracker. A Menstrual Symptoms Tracker is displayed in the appendix.

CHAPTER V
INFERTILITY AND ENDOMETRIOSIS

Even in its mildest form endometriosis can be associated with infertility. Clinical data from some studies indicate that the prevalence of infertility is about 15% in the general population. However, this approaches 30% to 50% in patients with endometriosis. Infertile women are 6 to 8 times more likely to have endometriosis than fertile women. Conservative surgical procedures such as laparoscopy and robotic laparoscopy for endometriosis are followed by subsequent pregnancies in at least half of the cases. This depends on the severity of the endometriosis.[1,2] It should be noted that, the notion that endometriosis causes infertility remains controversial. While a reasonable body of evidence demonstrates an association between endometriosis and infertility, a direct cause has not been clearly established.[2]

No mechanism has been identified to adequately explain the link between endometriosis, and subfertility. Several mechanisms have been proposed. However, none of these mechanisms have been proven to decrease infertility in women with endometriosis. The various mechanisms are: [2,3]

42 | INFERTILITY AND ENDOMETRIOSIS

- Distorted pelvic anatomy.
- Altered peritoneal environment.
- Altered systemic immune function.
- Endocrine and ovulatory abnormalities.
- Abnormal tubal function.
- Abnormal fertilization and implantation.
- Abnormal endometrial function.

Distorted Pelvic Anatomy

Significant pelvic adhesions, which includes those that are related or result from endometriosis, can impair oocyte release from the ovary or impede ovum pick up or transport. [2,3]

Altered Peritoneal Function

It has been shown that women with endometriosis have an increased volume of peritoneal fluid with increased peritoneal fluid concentrations of various inflammatory agents including prostaglandins and cytokines. These alterations may disrupt oocyte, sperm, embryo and fallopian tube function. [2,3]

Altered Systemic Immune Function

IgG and IgA antibodies and lymphocytes may be increased in the endometrium of women with endometriosis. These abnormalities may alter endometrial responsiveness and embryo implantation. [2,3]

Endocrine and Ovulatory Abnormalities

Numerous endocrine and ovulatory disorders may be present in women with endometriosis including the luteinized unruptured follicle syndrome, luteal phase dysfunction, abnormal follicular growth, and premature and multiple luteinizing hormone (LH) surges.[2,3]

Abnormal Utero-tubal Transport

Women with endometriosis may demonstrate a reduction in physiologic utero-tubal transport capacity compared to control subjects. [2,3] This may be a factor with proximal tubal blockage in some patients with endometriosis without any other obvious causes.

Abnormal Fertilization and Implantation

In women with endometriosis, it is not clear, if abnormal fertilization and implantation contribute to decreased fertility. [2,3]

Impaired Implantation

Some evidence suggests that disorders of endometrial function may contribute to the increase in infertility. A reduced endometrial cell adhesion molecule during the time of implantation has been described in some women with endometriosis.

Other observations support the concept that endometriosis may represent one component of a disease. A disease that is characterized by dysfunction in multiple components of the genital tract, including the cervix, endometrium, fallopian tubes, and peritoneum. [2,3]

Management of Infertility

The clinical management of one who has endometriosis and infertility should be individualized. The age of the patient must be considered as well as the duration of infertility, medical history, pelvic pain and the stage of endometriosis, male factor, and family history.

44 | INFERTILITY AND ENDOMETRIOSIS

Medical Treatment: There is no evidence that medical treatment of endometriosis in infertile women improves fertility. A study comparing medical therapy to no treatment was essentially equivalent. In a review of several studies utilizing ovulation suppressive agents (progestins, danazol, GnRH agonists), in an effort to improve fertility in women with endometriosis, there was no apparent benefit to use of ovulation suppression medication. The use of ovulation suppression agents increased the time to conceive. The exception was the use of GnRH agonist for suppression of endometriosis in patients undergoing IVF. Using a GnRH agonist for 3-6 months prior to IVF was found to increase clinical pregnancy and live birth rates.[4,5,6] It's plausible that similar results may be obtained with the newer GnRH antagonists.

Hormonal treatment is extremely effective in reducing pelvic pain associated with endometriosis, which may also improve sexual function (the frequency of intercourse) thereby increasing fertility. Hormone therapy may also be of value in the postoperative treatment of infertile women with endometriosis who are considering *in vitro* fertilization/embryo transfer (IVF/ET).[3]

Surgical Treatment: A thorough infertility evaluation should be initiated prior to surgery. The surgical management of endometriosis is based on redressing the extent of endometriosis and attempt, to normalize the anatomy. During surgery, the extent, of endometriosis should be ascertained, staged, and recorded. Photo and/or video documentation is advisable for the patient to view. To the fullest extent possible, endometriotic lesions should be either surgically excised or ablated/fulgurated. Deeply invasive endometriotic lesions should be surgically excised. Superficial peritoneal implants may be either ablated/fulgurated or surgically excised.[7,8] Endometriomas should be excised, with preservation of as much normal ovarian tissue as possible. Pelvic anatomy should be restored to normal, and all adhesions should be excised. Laparoscopy can be successfully used to treat almost all patients with endometriosis. Since a surgical procedure such as laparoscopy is used to diagnose endometriosis, it is recommended to render surgical treatment at the time of the initial diagnosis.[9] Acceptable pregnancy rates after laparoscopic surgery for endometriosis have been reported in women with mild to moderate disease. Surgical treatment with removal of endometrial implants has the potential benefit of decreasing inflammation which may improve fertility. In patients with severe disease potential benefits of surgery include lysis of adhesions and attempts at restoration of normal pelvic anatomy. Both have the added benefit of possibly abating pelvic pain.[9,10]

Combination Medical-surgical Therapy: Medical management for endometriosis consists of either preoperative or postoperative medical therapy. Preoperative therapy is reported to reduce pelvic vascularity and the size of endometriotic implants. This reduces intraoperative blood loss and decrease the amount of surgical resection needed. Postoperative medical therapy is advocated to eradicate residual endometriotic implants. This is applicable to patients with extensive disease in whom resection of all implants is impossible or inadvisable. Postoperative hormonal therapy has also been recommended to treat endometriosis that isn't visible (microscopic disease). Although theoretically advantageous, combination medical-surgical treatment has not consistently been shown to enhance fertility.[11,12]

46 | Infertility and Endometriosis

In summary, endometriosis is associated with infertility, even in its mildest forms. When formulating a management plan for patients with infertility and endometriosis, female age, duration of infertility, pelvic pain, and stage of endometriosis should be carefully considered.[4,11] It is also important to be mindful of the old adage that "one size does not fit all" when deciding on treatment.

Take Away

- Relevant to treatment, laparoscopic ablation, excision or fulguration has been shown to be beneficial, relevant to improving pregnancy rates in natural cycles.
- Medical treatment, per se has demonstrated marginal benefits for improving pregnancy rates.

Power Point`

Endometriosis has a profound impact on the quality of life, developing the optimal therapy that also improves fertility remains a challenge.

SECTION III

SPECIAL INTEREST

CHAPTER VI
FIBROID TUMORS AND ENDOMETRIOSIS

Fibroids are benign (non-cancerous) tumors, or growths that consist of smooth muscle cells and fibrous connective tissue. These growths originate within the muscle wall of the uterus. Each fibroid is thought to arise from a single cell which grows into a mass or group of masses. They range in size from as small as a grain of rice to as large as a melon. In some cases, fibroids can grow into the uterine cavity or outward from the uterine wall on stalks. Both estrogen and progesterone hormones (products of the ovaries) are thought to promote the growth of these tumors. Some tumors will remain stable in size over many years, while others will appear suddenly and grow rapidly. Whether or not treatment is needed depends on the size and location of the tumor, along with the rate of growth of the fibroids and whether they are symptomatic.

Symptoms are generally a consequence of the size and location of the fibroids themselves. Heaviness or pressure in the pelvis can be felt as pressure is placed on surrounding organs such as the bladder or large intestine, if the tumor protrudes into the endometrial cavity, heavy or irregular bleeding may occur. In 1 in 10,000 cases, a fibroid

50 | FIBROID TUMORS AND ENDOMETRIOSIS

may develop into a rare form of cancer (sarcoma). Sarcomas are a very aggressive form of cancer.

Parenthetically, many fibroids produce no symptoms at all. They are simply noted during routine annual examinations or when a pap smear is performed. Other fibroids will cause heavy and prolonged periods. In some situations, the size and position of the fibroid(s) may be responsible for pain, which can be related to periods, severe menstrual cramps or painful sex.[1,2,3]

An estimated 20% to 50% of women of reproductive age currently have fibroids. Additionally, up to 77% of women will develop fibroids sometime during their childbearing years. Only about one-third of these fibroids are large enough to be detected by an obstetrician-gynecologist during a pelvic exam, so they are often undiagnosed. In more than 99% of fibroid cases, the tumors are not cancerous and do not increase the risk for uterine cancer.

Endometriosis and uterine fibroids are common gynecological disorders in fertile women and are not mutually exclusive. Both can occur and cause problems at the same time. Uterine fibroids, as previously stated, are estimated to occur in 33-77% of women during their reproductive years. Even though most fibroids are asymptomatic, they are still the most common reason for hysterectomy. The symptoms are related to their size, number and location in the uterus. Common symptoms are menorrhagia, pelvic pressure, pain and urinary symptoms. The incidence of endometriosis is even more difficult to determine because, the exact diagnosis requires invasive intervention. In symptomatic women who have had surgery, the incidence has varied between 2 and 18%. The symptoms of endometriosis are chronic pelvic pain, dysmenorrhea, menorrhagia, dyspareunia and dysuria. A relevant study demonstrated that about 20% of patients with symptomatic fibroids also had endometriosis. On the other hand, 26% of patients with symptomatic endometriosis had fibroids. The prevalence of endometriosis and fibroids seemed to coincide, and they both were independent factors associated with subfertility. Additionally, the proportion of asymptomatic women is significant.[2,4]

It has been suggested that these two disorders may be associated with each other. Nevertheless, their etiologies do have some similarities. Both of these diseases are steroid hormone dependent, acting similarly under the influence of estrogen. In one study, women with uterine fibroids were reported to have endometriosis more often than those without fibroids.

It is common for women who present with fibroid tumors to complain of pelvic pain and severe cramps, along with a host of other endometriosis like symptoms. Regardless of the tumor size, fibroid tumors were stated to be the cause of the pain. In my experience, more often than not, endometriosis was the cause of the pain. It's safe to say one can have both endometriosis and fibroid tumors at the same time. Several years ago, one of my studies revealed 85% of women, who had 12-week size fibroids or greater and severe cyclic pelvic pain, had both fibroid tumors and endometriosis.[5,6]

Since fibroids and endometriosis can occur at the same time, if a person has fibroid tumors and experiences endometriosis-like symptoms, especially monthly pelvic pain/cramps before during or after menstruation, it's likely endometriosis is the cause of the pain, particularly if the pain occurs in the same location. In fact, I have seen hundreds of patients through the years, who had fibroids and endometriosis, where fibroid tumors were initially blamed for the pain.

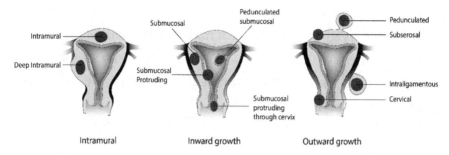

Figure 2. Various Types of fibroids and their locations

Table 5: Common Symptoms of Endometriosis and Fibroid Tumors[2,4]

Endometriosis Symptoms	Fibroid Symptoms
Pelvic pain	Pelvic pressure
Dysmenorrhea (painful periods)	Pelvic pain
Infertility	Enlargement of the lower abdomen
GI symptoms related to menses, (bloating, nausea and/or diarrhea)	Heavy menstrual bleeding, which can be heavy enough to cause anemia
Irregular or heavy menstrual bleeding	Frequent urination
Low back or leg pain related to menses	Difficulty emptying the bladder
Painful defecation during menses	Constipation
Painful intercourse	Painful intercourse

Diagnosis of Uterine Fibroids

In most cases, fibroids are diagnosed by the obstetrician and gynecologist during a pelvic examination. During the exam a fibroid is felt to be an enlarged irregular firm mass in the pelvis. Some tumors may be at the umbilicus (navel) or above it. The size of the uterus which contains the fibroid is estimated, based on the size of a comparable pregnancy.[2]

See Table 6

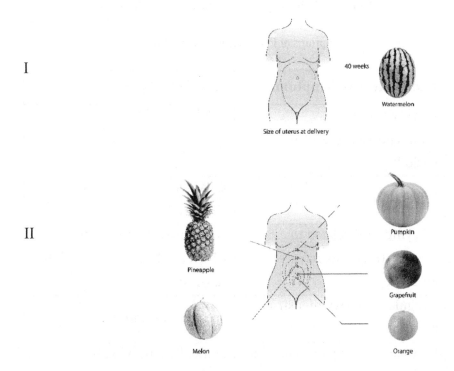

Figure 2

I. A pregnant uterus (40 weeks) is about the size of a watermelon.
II. Size comparison between fibroids and common fruit.

54 | FIBROID TUMORS AND ENDOMETRIOSIS

Table 6: Size Comparisons: Weeks of Pregnancy Versus Fruit[5]

Uterine Fibroid Weeks of Pregnancy	=	Fruit
Normal Uterus	=	Small Pear
10-Week Fibroid	=	Orange
12 -Week Fibroid	=	Grapefruit
16- Week Fibroid	=	Melon
22-Week Fibroid	=	Pineapple
28-Week Fibroid	=	Pumpkin

Ultrasound is the best method for determining the size, location, and number of fibroids in a uterus. It is usually advantageous to perform ultrasound on all patients with fibroids because determining the exact size and location of fibroids is often difficult with a pelvic examination alone. Other imaging such as **magnetic resonance imaging (MRI)** can show the size and location of fibroids in more detail. MRI can also aid in the identification of different types of tumors, which can help determine appropriate treatment options. An MRI is often used in women with a larger uterus. **Sonohysterography**, also called a saline infusion sonogram, is the utilization of saline to expand the uterine cavity, making it easier to obtain images of submucosal fibroids and the lining of the uterus, particularly, in women who have heavy menstrual bleeding or are attempting to get pregnant. On the other hand, **Hysteroscopy** uses a small, lighted telescope called a hysteroscope, which is inserted through the cervix into the uterus with saline. The saline expands the uterine cavity and allows for visual evaluation of the inside of the uterus.[5]

Treatment

There is no single best approach to uterine fibroid treatment. The treatment must be individualized based on symptoms, extent of disease and patient preferences. There are many treatment options available. Many women with uterine fibroids experience no signs or symptoms, while others experience mild, annoying symptoms that they can tolerate and live with. In such cases watchful waiting may be the best option. This is especially true since fibroids are non-cancerous and rarely interfere with pregnancy. Fibroids tend to grow slowly or not at all and often shrink after menopause, when levels of reproductive hormones drop. However, for symptomatic patients or those desiring management, the following options are available:

Medication for Uterine Fibroids

Medications for uterine fibroids generally target hormones that regulate the menstrual cycle, with a particular focus on heavy menstrual bleeding and pelvic pressure. However, these medications don't eliminate fibroids. Gonadotropin-releasing hormone (GnRH) antagonist and gonadotropin-releasing hormone agonist (GnRH) are frequency used and may shrink them. Shrinkage may occur while on the medication. The tumors may resume growth once the medication is discontinued. Other commonly used medications include oral contraceptives.[7,8]

Oral contraceptives are the first-line medical treatments for most fibroid symptoms, although the quality of evidence for their use or positive results is low. Injectable long-acting gonadotropin-releasing hormone (GnRH) agonists (leuprolide acetate) are effective, but their use is limited by hypoestrogenic side effects. Alternative medical treatment options include the administration of additional hormonal therapy to mitigate side effects. New oral GnRH antagonists (elagolix and relugolix), administered with estradiol and norethindrone acetate, have been shown to reduce heavy menstrual bleeding, pelvic pain and anemia in women with uterine fibroids. They are approved for the treatment of uterine fibroids for up to 24 months.[6] These same GnRH antagonists (elagolix and relugolix), combined with estradiol and norethindrone acetate are also being studied for treatment of pelvic pain associated with endometriosis. [7,8,9,10]

Surgery for Uterine Fibroids

Uterine artery embolization (UAE) involves the injection of small particles into the arteries supplying the uterus. The procedure is done on an outpatient basis by an interventional radiologist, whereby a small incision is made in the top of the leg where it meets the pelvis. A catheter is then inserted into an artery in the leg, which is passed into the arteries that supply blood to the uterus. Small plastic or gelatin particles are then inserted into the arteries through the catheter, which stick to the vessel walls causing a clot to develop and blocking off the blood supply. Once the blood supply is cut off, the fibroids shrink and degenerate. UAE is an effective treatment for shrinking fibroids and relieving the symptoms they cause. Studies have shown that 3 out of 4 women who undergo UAE experience relief from fibroid symptoms. However, 1 out of 5 women who have undergone UAE may require another surgery, including a second UAE, myomectomy or hysterectomy for their fibroids due to complications such as severe pain.[10]

Hysteroscopic myomectomy may be indicated if the fibroids are contained inside the uterine cavity, (submucosal). The procedure is carried out by placing a small, lighted telescope through the cervix into the uterus. Saline is injected to expand the uterine cavity, which allows the gynecologist to visually evaluate the inside of the uterus and, sometimes, to remove part or all of the submucosal fibroids.[10]

Radiofrequency ablation is a procedure in which radiofrequency energy is used to destroy uterine fibroids by debilitating the blood vessels that feed them. This can be done during a laparoscopic or transcervical procedure. A similar procedure called cryomyolysis freezes the fibroids. An Yttrium Aluminum Garnet (YAG) laser or Carbon Dioxide (CO_2) laser can also be used via laparoscopy to drill extensively into fibroid tumors (myolysis), which damages and impedes the blood supply to the fibroids tumors, and causes shrinkage and reduction in fibroid symptoms.[11, 12]

Laparoscopic or robotic myomectomy is performed by placing a thin, lighted telescope-like instrument in the abdomen through a small incision. The abdomen is then inflated with CO_2 gas, which allows for the pelvis and abdominal cavity to be viewed on a monitor using a small camera attached to one of the instruments. Special instruments are used to perform surgical procedures such as myomectomy or the removal of fibroids. Robotic myomectomy may allow for better magnification, and 3D visualization of the pelvis, which could lead to a better outcome. However, the number of incisions made on the abdomen is increased. Fortunately, endometriosis can be diagnosed and surgically treated while laparoscopy is being carried out to perform a myomectomy.[4,13,14]

58 | FIBROID TUMORS AND ENDOMETRIOSIS

Abdominal or laparotomy myomectomy is used if there are multiple very large fibroids deeply embedded into the uterine wall, an open vertical or horizontal abdominal surgical incision may be indicated to remove the fibroids.

It is also possible to diagnosis and treat endometriosis while performing abdominal myomectomy. Risks associated with abdominal myomectomy are blood loss and increased risk of scar tissue formation which may necessitate blood transfusion and hospitalization for one to three days. [13, 15, 16]

Hysterectomy is the surgical removal of the uterus and is the only treatment that prevents fibroids from recurring. It is a last-resort treatment for women who do not wish to preserve their fertility. The procedure is usually recommended for women with fibroids that cause pain and heavy menstrual bleeding, which interfere with daily life. It is an option for those who do not desire or are unsatisfied with medical treatment. However, it is advisable to commence treatment with medical options before resorting to this procedure.

There are several ways to perform a hysterectomy, depending on the size, number, and location of the fibroids. The procedure can be rendered via an open procedure; laparoscopy, robotic laparoscopy, or vaginally.[16,17] The type of procedure should be decided in consultation with the surgeon performing the procedure. Consideration should be given to whether the ovaries are removed, as this may cause surgical menopause, and whether the fallopian tubes are removed, as this may reduce the risk of ovarian cancer.

Table 7: Surgical Treatment of Fibroids and Possibly Endometriosis [14,19,18,21,22,23]

Procedure	Fibroid Impairment	Fibroid Removal	Uterus Removal	Endometriosis can be diagnosed & treated
Uterine Artery Embolization	√			
Hysteroscopic Myomectomy		√		
Radiofrequency Ablation	√			√
Laparoscopic Myomectomy		√		√
Abdominal Myomectomy		√		√
Hysterectomy			√	√

In summary fibroids can be of different sizes and located in different areas of the uterus. Women may experience varying symptoms, or in some cases no symptoms at all. Endometriosis also presents in different ways, has various classifications, and is associated with multiple symptoms. Therefore, it is reasonable to conclude that, given the two problems and their many variations, patients will have different treatment preferences and options. Thus, the care or treatment plan for each patient must be individualized. [4,14]

Take Away

- Tailored treatment plans should be considered for patients who have both fibroids and endometriosis.
- Treatment plans should be made jointly with the patient and physician.
- New medications (GnRH antagonists), elagolix, and relugolix, can be used to treat heavy menstrual bleeding associated with fibroids.
- New medications (GnRH antagonists), elagolix, and relugolix, can be used to treat pelvic pain associated with endometriosis.

Power Point

The GnRH antagonists (elagolix and relugolix) may prevent the need for surgery, particularly hysterectomy in patients with both fibroids and endometriosis.

CHAPTER VII
ADENOMYOSIS AND ENDOMETRIOSIS

Adenomyosis, is a benign condition in which the glands of the endometrium (the lining of the uterine cavity) infiltrate the myometrium (muscle wall of the uterus). Adenomyosis has long been regarded as a close cousin of endometriosis. As previously, stated endometriosis is a benign disorder where the endometrial glands can be found outside of the uterus in other parts of the body, such as the ovaries, fallopian tubes, cul de sac and appendix. Adenomyosis can cause pelvic pain, severe menstrual cramps, and lower abdominal pressure in addition, bloating and heavy prolonged menstrual bleeding.[1]

The condition presents most commonly as a diffuse disease involving the entire myometrium. It can also present in a focal area of the uterus, known as an adenomyoma. Additionally, adenomyosis can be associated with other conditions such as fibroids, endometrial polyps, and as previously stated endometriosis. In fact, many of the symptoms applicable to endometriosis are like those found in adenomyosis. Beyond this an MRI study noted that the prevalence of endometriosis in adenomyosis patients was 80.6 %. The prevalence of adenomyosis in endometriosis patients was 91.1 %. [2,3] The adenomyotic lesions generally develop in the median region of the upper two-thirds of the uterine wall.[2] Undoubtedly there is a high association of adenomyosis with endometriosis and vice versa. Furthermore, the establishment of the clinical diagnosis of adenomyosis is difficult, because the presenting symptoms are commonly found in other disorders. A homogeneously enlarged (globular) uterus on pelvic examination is suggestive of the diagnosis of adenomyosis along with MRI imaging.

Adenomyosis is said to be commonly found or diagnosed in middle-aged women and women who had children. About 80% of the cases occur in women at 40-50 years old and 90% in women who have had children. Some studies also suggest that women who have had prior uterine surgery may be at risk for adenomyosis. Though the cause of adenomyosis isn't known, studies have suggested that various hormones, including estrogen, progesterone, prolactin, and follicle stimulating hormone may trigger the condition. [2]

Table 8: Adenomyosis and Endometriosis Symptoms and Location [4,5]

Disorder	Location	Symptoms
Adenomyosis	Glands in the myometrium of the uterus	Pelvic pain, menstrual cramps, heavy prolonged menstrual bleeding, pelvic pressure, and bloating
Endometriosis	Glands outside of the uterus, may be found in the	Pelvic pain, menstrual cramps, irregular or heavy

	ovaries, bowels, fallopian tubes, appendix	menstrual bleeding, infertility, painful intercourse, low back pain, painful defecation

Diagnosing Adenomyosis

Until recently, the only definitive way to diagnose adenomyosis was to perform a hysterectomy, where the uterine tissue would be examined under a microscope to confirm the diagnosis. However, thanks to imaging technology, it is now possible to recognize adenomyosis without surgery. Magnetic resonance imaging (MRI) or transvaginal ultrasound can be used to appreciate the characteristics or extent of the disease in the uterus.[5,6]

Transvaginal ultrasound. If adenomyosis, is suspected a pelvic examination may reveal an enlarged boggy and tender uterus. Transvaginal ultrasound can allow visualization of the uterus, endometrium, and myometrium. Although ultrasound cannot definitively diagnose adenomyosis, it can be helpful in ruling out other conditions with similar symptoms.[5]

Magnetic resonance imaging (MRI) is a medical imaging technique that uses a magnetic field and computer-generated radio waves to create detailed images of the organs and tissues. Fortunately, MRI can be used to confirm a diagnosis of adenomyosis in women with abnormal uterine bleeding.[5]

Treatment of Adenomyosis

Medication for Adenomyosis

Medical treatments for adenomyosis follows the principles of the management of endometriosis which are usually aimed at reducing the production of one's own estrogen along with inducing endometrial modification with progestins. Clinical evidence points to the clear and harmful effect of uninterrupted ovulatory cycles on the development and persistence of adenomyosis. The objectives of medical treatment are to inhibit ovulation and eliminate menstruation. Medical therapies commonly used in the treatment of adenomyosis, like those for endometriosis include gonadotropin-releasing hormone agonist (GnRH agonist), gonadotropin-releasing hormone antagonist (GnRH antagonist), oral contraceptives (OCs), progestins, danazol, and aromatase inhibitors (AI). These agents create a decrease in estrogen (GnRH agonists, GnRH antagonists, AIs), increase in androgens (danazol) while others increase progesterone (OCs, progestins) environment, with suppression of endometrial cell proliferation. However, medical treatments are symptomatic, and lesions may survive the use of any drug, at any dose, and for any length of time, which is a factor that allows resumption of their past activity at treatment discontinuation.[7,8]

Medical treatments may represent standard therapies for endometriosis and some such as GnRH agonists and antagonists are associated with adverse events that impact their long-term use and adherence. The issues are hypoestrogenemia or decreased estrogen which can cause hot flushes and insomnia. Additionally, accelerated bone demineralization or bone loss which may not be reversable.

Since no medical treatment for endometriosis is universally effective, it should be emphasized that this concept is also applicable to adenomyosis therapy. However, keep in mind that there are several consequential clinical studies that are germane to new drug development that are applicable to endometriosis and would probably be applicable to the medical treatment of adenomyosis.[8,9]

Surgery for Adenomyosis

Uterine Artery Embolization (UAE). UAE has been used to treat symptomatic fibroids since the 1990s, and now there is increasing evidence to suggest that it is also effective in the treatment of adenomyosis.[10]

High Intensity Focused Ultrasound (HIFU). HIFU is another minimally invasive treatment that focuses high intensity ultrasound on the target lesion, causing coagulative necrosis and shrinkage of the lesion. Both MRI and ultrasound can be used for guidance for the procedure. Ultrasound guided HIFU was shown to be technically successful in up to 94.6% of patients in a review of 2,549 patients with symptomatic adenomyosis.[11]

Endometrial ablation. The procedure involves destruction of the lining of the uterus by inserting of an energy source such as electrocautery, heated **balloon therapy,** or **radiofrequency ablation, or microwave ablation** into the uterine cavity. The procedure has been found to be effective in relieving symptoms such as heavy prolonged menstrual bleeding in some patients where adenomyosis hasn't penetrated deeply into the myometrium of the uterus. However, the

66 | ADENOMYOSIS AND ENDOMETRIOSIS

procedure should only be done on women who do not plan to have children in the future.[10, 11,12]

Adenomyomectomy. (Laparoscopy and Laparotomy). Adenomyomectomy, is the resection or removal of adenomyosis from the uterus. It can be performed via laparoscopy or laparotomy. Focal adenomyosis resection can be performed using laparotomy or laparoscopy whereas diffuse adenomyosis is limited to using laparotomy. Laparoscopy can be used for treating focal adenomyosis, although it entails a risk of leaving some of the lesions unexcised. [10,11] Laparoscopy is also used in conjunction with laparotomy for treating diffuse adenomyosis. Both procedures increase the risk of uterine rupture. For example, pregnancies occurring in women who have been treated for uterine adenomyosis have a higher risk of spontaneous rupture than those without a history of surgery. A review suggested that the risk of uterine rupture after uterine adenomyosis is 6.0%. Additionally, the risk of uterine rupture due to pregnancy after removal of uterine adenomyosis is >1.0%, compared to 0.26% in pregnancies following myomectomy.[12,13,14, 15]

Hysterectomy. Is the definitive treatment option for intractable symptomatic adenomyosis when medical or other conservative treatments have failed to control the symptoms. The procedure can be performed via laparotomy, laparoscopy, robotic laparoscopy or vaginally.[16] Once a decision to proceed with hysterectomy has been made, the possibility of oophorectomy should be discussed. In general, it is not considered necessary to routinely remove the ovaries in premenopausal women. However, it may be indicated in women who suffer from cyclical symptoms, with concomitant ovarian endometriosis or those who are considered to have an increased risk of developing ovarian cancer, including those with a family history of the condition.[18]A recent study suggested that the risk of developing ovarian cancer in women with newly diagnosed adenomyosis is increased by 4-5-fold. If the finding is confirmed, there is a strong case to consider prophylactic salpingooophorectomy at the time of hysterectomy for adenomyosis in premenopausal women.[19,20,21]

Endometriosis, and adenomyosis does occur together. According to one study, the prevalence of endometriosis in patients with adenomyosis was 80.6 % while the prevalence of adenomyosis in patients with endometriosis was 91.1 %. The awareness that adenomyosis and endometriosis are two problems that can have similar symptoms and can occur in the same patient at the same time is extremely important for optimal management of an afflicted patient. In view of this, it's imperative that each patient receive a tailored care plan or patient-centered care.

Take Away

Custom treatment plans should be considered for patients who have both adenomyosis and endometriosis.

CHAPTER VIII
CANCER AND ENDOMETRIOSIS

Aside from concerns such as debilitating pelvic pain, infertility, and quality of life issues, women with endometriosis often grapple with the proverbial questions such as "can endometriosis turn into cancer?" "Does having endometriosis increase the risk of getting cancer or is endometriosis a type of cancer?" In response to these concerning questions. Endometriosis is benign. However, it shares some characteristics similar, to invasive cancer, such as peritoneal implants, local invasion, and distant metastasis. Although endometriosis cannot be termed a premalignant condition or turn into cancer, data suggest that endometriosis does have malignant potential. In fact, women with endometriosis are at increased risk not only of ovarian cancer, but possibly endometrial, breast cancer, melanoma, and non-Hodgkin's lymphoma. Additionally, evidence suggests that endometriosis especially ovarian endometriotic cyst, may be produced from a single cell or by clones of a single cell, which can yield abnormal growth with premalignant potential. Therefore, the risk of development of ovarian and other cancers related to endometriosis cannot be ignored.[1,2]

Endometriosis and Associated Cancers

Ovarian Cancer

The prevalence of endometriosis-associated ovarian cancer varies depending on the subtype of ovarian cancer. A review of several studies found that endometriotic-associated carcinoma was most commonly seen in clear cell carcinoma, followed by endometrioid carcinoma, serous carcinoma, and mucinous carcinoma. The study concludes that endometriotic cells may undergo changes that lead to malignant potential.

Although endometriosis is considered a benign disease, the risk of developing ovarian cancer is slightly higher in endometriosis patients compared to the general population, with a relative risk ranging from 1.3 to 1.9%. Two mechanisms have been suggested to explain this correlation: shared risk factors and effects, and the gradual transformation of endometriotic cells into cancer cells. Atypical endometriosis is considered an intermediate state between endometriosis and ovarian cancer and is possible precancerous condition, with more than two-thirds of endometriosis-related ovarian tumors developing in the presence of atypical endometriosis.

Risk factors for the development of atypical endometriosis include early age of onset and long duration of disease, as well as obesity, dysmenorrhea, perimenopause, and menopause. In addition, irregular vaginal bleeding, tumor fixation during a gynecological examination, a tumor diameter over 9 cm, a rapid increase in tumor size, uterine fibroids, thyroid disease, and multiple foci of endometriosis are also considered risk factors. Endometriosis and ovarian cancer also share similar features, such as local invasion, propensity for new blood vessel formation, and resistance to the mechanism of cell death.[3,4]

The most important conclusions reached by the studies are the following:

- Ovarian endometriosis is a risk factor that can lead to the development of endometrioid and clear cell ovarian carcinomas.
- The risk of malignant transformation varies between 2 and 17%.
- Risk factors for endometriosis associated ovarian cancer are ovarian endometrioma ≥ 9 cm, in peri- and post-menopausal patients.
- Endometriosis associated ovarian cancer patients are 10 years younger than other ovarian cancer patients.
- Hyperestrogenemia, is a risk factor for the development of endometriosis-associated ovarian cancer. Endometriosis associated ovarian cancer presents with some specific clinical features that distinguish it from ovarian cancer. It affects younger patients, shows lower CA-125 levels, and has a better prognosis. Additionally, there is a higher number of clear cells than in ovarian cancer. The relative risk of developing specific subtypes of ovarian cancer for patients with endometriosis is calculated as follows:
- Clear cell ovarian carcinoma - 3.05
- Endometrioid ovarian carcinoma - 2.04
- Low-grade serous ovarian carcinoma - 2.11
- High-grade serous ovarian carcinoma - 1.13
- Mucinous ovarian carcinoma - 1.02

72 | CANCER AND ENDOMETRIOSIS

An extensive and significant survey compared the endometriosis associated ovarian cancer, with the non-endometriosis associated ovarian cancer and reached the following conclusions: [5,6,7]

- Endometriosis increases the risk of ovarian cancer.
- Endometriosis associated ovarian cancer patients have better prognosis and survival.
- Endometriosis associated ovarian cancer are more common in nulliparous women (women who has never given birth).
- Endometrioid and clear cell subtypes are more common in endometriosis associated ovarian cancer, while serous carcinomas are less frequent.

Apart from the indisputable evidence of the association of endometriosis with ovarian carcinoma, other factors reduce the risk of ovarian cancer in women with endometriosis. Since 2004, oral contraceptives have been shown to reduce the risk of ovarian cancer. By 50–60% in women with endometriosis. Studies published in 2013 established that unilateral oophorectomy significantly reduces the risk of ovarian cancer compared to endometriosis patients who underwent conservative nonsurgical treatment. Additionally, the studies reported on the protective effect of childbirth and hysterectomy. The available data considered so far indisputably prove that endometriosis is associated with the development of some ovarian cancer subtypes. Regarding the location of endometriosis an intriguing question is whether there is a link between the location of endometriosis and the risk of cancer. It should be noted that not only is the extent or stage of endometriosis important, but the location is also consequential. The results of a published 2018 study covered the period of 1987 to 2012 and included 49,933 women with surgically verified endometriosis, are as follows depending on the organ localization of endometriosis, the distribution is as follows: [5]

- Ovaries - 51%
- Peritoneum - 44%
- Deep infiltrating endometriosis - 5%

It should also be noted that endometriosis may have been found in one or all three locations in the same patient at the same time.

The study shows that patients with endometriosis have a 2.3 times higher risk of developing ovarian cancer, wherein endometriosis associated ovarian cancer are primarily endometrioid and clear cell sub-types. In addition, the study showed that endometriosis patients have a significant risk of developing borderline ovarian tumors. Depending on the localization of endometriosis, ovarian cancer risk is highest among women with ovarian endometriosis, while peritoneal and deep infiltrating endometriosis do not increase the risk.[7,8] After a 10-year follow-up, the authors found that the excess risk of ovarian cancer, among women with ovarian endometriosis translates into two excess cases per 1,000 patients.

It was noted that the following clinical groups are at an increased risk of developing endometriosis-associated ovarian cancer: patients aged > 45 years; nulliparous patients, postmenopausal women with a diagnosis of endometriosis; patients with endometriomas ≥ 9 cm and those with hypoestrogenism. The frequency of endometriosis associated ovarian cancer varies between 2 and 17%, and endometrioid and clear cell ovarian carcinomas are the most common. Only ovarian endometriosis (not peritoneal and deep infiltrating endometriosis) is related to the progression of endometriosis-associated ovarian cancer and malignant transformation progresses to atypical endometriosis. Although endometriosis-associated ovarian cancer has a good prognosis, adequate follow-up and monitoring after treatment are recommended.[9,10,11]

Breast Cancer

The potential association between endometriosis and breast cancer remains unclear, although the issue is of particular importance given the relatively high incidence of both conditions. Even a minor increase in breast cancer risk would have a major clinical impact. It is important to keep in mind the impact that hormonal medical treatment may have on breast cancer risk, as opposed to endometriosis itself.[12] Beyond this the risk for breast cancer was increased among women aged $\geq$ 50 years at first diagnosis of endometriosis.[13] Whether or not one has endometriosis, it is important for women to check their breasts regularly. Make sure to seek medical assistance if irregularities are noted. No one can discern changes in their body as well as the person who is in the body.[12]

Endometrial Cancer

The relationship between endometriosis and endometrial carcinoma is potentially interesting because it could suggest a baseline genetic predisposition of the endometrium of some women to undergo malignant transformation. An excess risk was also observed for endometrial cancer.[13] However, in population-based studies, no association has been found between endometriosis and endometrial carcinoma.[14]

Non-Hodgkin's Lymphoma

Some of the largest population-based studies have independently documented an association with non-Hodgkin lymphoma. However statistically significant results from various studies are based on a small number of observed cases. Thus, there is a cogent need for further confirmation. Potential explanations for an increase in risk of non-Hodgkin lymphoma in women with endometriosis are currently speculative.[15]

Melanoma

The largest and most comprehensive analysis of endometriosis and skin cancer to date supports an association between a personal history of endometriosis and skin cancer risk. It also suggests that the association is most pronounced for cutaneous melanoma. It is still unclear whether common associated factors between the two diseases or systemic changes explain the observed associations between endometriosis and melanoma. Further research is needed to elucidate common pathways between these two diseases. Thus, the evidence is not yet conclusive. However, don't forget to cover up and have routine skin checks at your, annual physical.[16]

Other Cancers and Endometriosis

Investigations of associations with other cancers have been sparse. Consequently, no firm conclusion can be drawn regarding subsequent risk of other malignancies in women with endometriosis.[17]

76 | CANCER AND ENDOMETRIOSIS

Table 9: Cancer in Women with Endometriosis[1]

Cancer	% of Women with Endo who have Cancer	% of General Population (US & Canada) with Cancer
Non-Hodgkin's Lymphoma	0.05%	0.02%
Ovarian Cancer	0.2%	0.04%
Breast Cancer	0.6%	0.1%
Melanoma	0.8%	0.01%

Reducing risks of cancer: Half of cancers are preventable, and there are several key actions that can be taken to lower one's risk. In general, to improve health and lower risk of cancer, try to have a balanced diet, limit alcohol intake, exercise regularly, maintain a healthy weight, and do not smoke. If you detect any changes in your body or symptoms that worry you, seek medical help immediately.

With all the other issues and problems confronting a woman with endometriosis, cancer and endometriosis should probably be low on the list of concerns. However, you should become concerned about the possibility of cancer in your own case, particularly, if sudden, unexpected, or otherwise unexplainable changes occur in your endometriosis symptoms. Pain is the most common symptom and abrupt increase in pain, continuous pain or pain that begins after menopause is an indication of concern. A comparatively rapid increase in size of an endometriotic mass or implant, hyperplasia change, as well as a change to an unusual appearance or rupture of an endometriotic cyst, should alert your gynecologist to the possibility of cancer.

Gynecologists should be very careful in recommending estrogen replacement therapy to patients with a history of endometriosis, due to the link between estrogens and endometrial cancer. A woman with endometriosis has more to risk than other patients who might receive estrogen replacement as she not only has her intrauterine endometrium to worry about but also endometriotic implants that are also subject to the effects of estrogen. Even postmenopausal women and women who have had hysterectomies and women who had removal of the ovaries, and who have a history of endometriosis should carefully consider the option to take estrogen, since it may activate both microscopic areas of endometriosis and cancer. Individualization is necessary due to the risk of osteoporosis associated with the lack of estrogen.

Although cancer developing from endometriosis is very rare, it does occur. Therefore, every woman with endometriosis should carefully monitor her symptoms and report any unusual, unexplainable change in symptoms to her gynecologist. All gynecologists should be cautious and thorough in diagnosing and treating their patients with endometriosis. Although cancer developing from endometriosis is rare, its potential cannot be taken lightly since the consequences of ignoring the possibility can be quite serious. [12,18,19]

Take Away

- There is no evidence that endometriosis causes cancer.
- There is no increase in overall incidence, of cancer in women with endometriosis.
- Women who have endometriosis of the ovary have an increased risk of ovarian cancer.
- Women with endometriosis have an increased risk of some malignancies, particularly ovarian cancer. The risk increases with early diagnosed or long-standing disease. Hysterectomy may have a preventive effect against ovarian cancer particularly if the ovaries and fallopian tubes are removed.[4]

Power Point

Most women with endometriosis never develop ovarian cancer. While some studies suggest a slightly increased risk of ovarian cancer, overall evidence indicates a low likelihood of developing the disease. Therefore, it is important to be, aware of the potential association between endometriosis and ovarian cancer, but there is no need to for excessive worry.

CHAPTER IX
RACE AND ENDOMETRIOSIS

Undoubtedly, endometriosis can occur in women of any race. However early theories proposed that the incidence of endometriosis was highest or occurred only in White women.[1] This assumption was based on stereotypes about race and class, despite the fact that the medical literature has been shown to be systematically flawed.[2,3] Many studies for example were not controlled for confounding variables such as cultural differences, childbearing patterns, availability of health care and attitudes towards menses and pain.[4] Understandably, the biases already created are problematic because they are difficult to resolve. In fact, such biases may still hinder the quality of care that some women receive even today.[2,3,5]

For completeness, it is important to discuss and connect the history of endometriosis in Black women and the social determinants of health (SDOH) and their relationship to better understand, "race and endometriosis,"[5,6] For example, in 1906, American sociologist W.E.B. Du Bois noted that social conditions, not genetics, impacted the health of Blacks and were responsible for racial disparities in mortality rates.[7] In 2010, the federal government formally recognized that social conditions, specifically the social determinants of health, were responsible for racial health disparities.[8,9] Therefore it is

80 | RACE AND ENDOMETRIOSIS

crucial to consider SDOH such as poverty, racism, access to healthcare, and other factors when examining the incidence and impact of endometriosis in Black women.

Today, the mainstream belief among scientists is that race is a social construct without biological meaning. In fact, the American Medical Association (AMA) adopted policies in 2020 that encouraged characterizing race as a social construct, rather than an inherent biological trait. The AMA also supported ending the practice of using race as a proxy for biology in medical education, research and clinical practice.[10]

Regarding the history of endometriosis and race, particularly among Black women, Dr. Frank Lloyd an African American Indianapolis physician reported in his 1964 study of 803 Black and White private major gynecological surgical patients, that there were 108 cases of endometriosis giving an overall incidence of 7.43 per cent. Of the 500 White patients 74 had endometriosis with an incidence of 7.7%, while 34 of the 234 Black patients had endometriosis with an incidence of 6.9%. He concluded that the incidence of endometriosis in Black patients may approach that seen in White patients.[11,12]

In 1976 another African American Gynecologist, Dr. Donald Chatman, published a seminal assessment of the negative impact of racial bias on patient care. Dr. Chatman noted that one in five of his private African American patients demonstrated laparoscopic evidence of endometriosis and 40 per cent of these women had been wrongly diagnosed with pelvic inflammatory disease (PID), which implied that they had been exposed to sexually transmitted diseases. He argued that these misdiagnoses stemmed from the still pervasive myth that women of color were somehow immune to endometriosis, aligned with the stereotype that African American women were more promiscuous than their White peers. Only by addressing racial biases regarding endometriosis and pelvic pain can African American women receive quality reproductive care.[2,3,13]

Amazingly, a contemporary study noted that African American women are only about half as likely to be diagnosed with endometriosis as compared to White women. The same review noted that Asian women were more than 50% more likely to have this diagnosis than White women. Also, the prevalence of endometriosis appears to be influenced by race/ethnicity.[14,15] Compared to White women, Black women were significantly less likely to be diagnosed with endometriosis.[16] The same held true for Hispanic women. However, Asian women were much more likely to have this diagnosis as opposed to White women. The investigators noted there is scant literature, assessing the influence of race/ethnicity on symptomatology, treatment access, preference, and response. Nonetheless, "Race/ethnicity may influence one's ability to access healthcare, which can impact appropriate management of endometriosis via a combination of socioeconomic and genetic influences.[17, 18]

In the studies of women based on surgical or self-reported diagnosis of endometriosis, there was a significantly decreased odds of the diagnosis of endometriosis in Black women compared to White women. However, in women presenting with infertility, there was no meaningful difference in endometriosis rates between White and Black women. Furthermore, the likelihood of diagnosis of endometriosis in Black compared to White women was similar in studies conducted before 1990 and those after 1990.

82 | RACE AND ENDOMETRIOSIS

For Asian women, there was no significant difference in endometriosis frequency, particularly when the diagnosis was self-reported, compared to White women. However, the chances of diagnosis of endometriosis in Asian women versus White women, were greater in studies published before compared to studies published after 1990. Because the chief presenting symptomatology of endometriosis often includes pelvic pain which may be influenced by psychosocial factors, women of various ethnic and cultural backgrounds likely have distinct clinical presentations. "The results suggest the likelihood of endometriosis diagnosis among women of different ethnicities is often partially influenced by the mode of diagnosis.[18,19]

External factors may also affect the diagnosis of endometriosis, as it can take 4 to 11 years before a diagnosis is made. There may be a residual implicit bias among healthcare professionals that the diagnosis is less likely in Black women. Additionally, newer literature indicates that race/ethnicity may influence disease severity; for example, Asian women are more likely to be diagnosed with stage III/IV endometriosis compared to White women.

The study found and reported that "there is currently little effort in the literature to explore the diagnostic journey for women with endometriosis through a culturally sensitive lens." Clinicians are encouraged to provide culturally sensitive care to the women they treat, as women of different ethnicities may present with varying symptomatology.

To find a solution to resolve such biases, it is necessary to recognize that endometriosis can occur in women of any race. Additionally, women of various ethnicities may present with different symptoms of endometriosis and may express different treatment preferences.[22]

There should be a plan to increase the number of Black and minority women's health professionals. Furthermore, research in endometriosis should shift focus from prevalence studies to examining patient symptoms and experiences, using verified and culturally sensitive patient outcome measurements.[23] It is also essential to advocate for an adaptation of an individualized and patient-centered approach to the management of endometriosis. This approach is necessary to achieve more accurate and timely diagnoses, and to enhance patient care.[3]

Take Away

- It is necessary to recognize that endometriosis can occur in women of any race.
- It is suggested that endometriosis may be less common amongst Black and Hispanic women, compared to White women. However, it is imperative to recognize the significant methodological flaws and bias driving the studies performed to date.[24]

Power Point

- In theory save for the social determinants of health (SDOH), which can contribute to many consequential ills, "all of us are essentially in the same biological boat."
- As previously stated, Black and Hispanic women may be at greater risk for endometriosis, due to exposure to toxins from hair products and the toxins in their neighborhood. [25,17,26]

CHAPTER X
UNNECESSARY HYSTERECTOMIES

Hysterectomy is the surgical procedure that involves removal of the uterus, and in some cases, the ovaries and other reproductive organs may also be removed. It is the most commonly performed major gynecological surgery in the United States, with over 400,000 procedures performed annually. Despite a progressive decrease in the number of hysterectomies performed in the US over the past few years, it is estimated that one in three women will have had a hysterectomy by age 60 years. Notably over 68% of benign hysterectomies performed in the United States are done for the primary indications of abnormal uterine bleeding, uterine fibroids, and endometriosis.[1]

Remarkably, a 2015 study published in the American Journal of Obstetrics and Gynecology provides evidence that alternatives to hysterectomy are underutilized, particularly in women undergoing hysterectomy for abnormal uterine bleeding, uterine fibroids, endometriosis, or pelvic pain. The study found that the rate of

86 | UNNECESSARY HYSTERECTOMIES

unsupportive pathology when hysterectomies were done for these indications was 18%, indicating that these procedures were unnecessary.[2]

Regarding the issue with the 2015 study, one of the primary reasons for the unnecessary hysterectomies was the failure to give alternatives. Additionally, the study, like others exposed disparities related to alternatives. The difficulty with disparities was highlighted, as White women were more likely than Black women and women classified as neither Black nor White to receive alternative treatment,[3,4] despite considering parity, body mass index, insurance, and other common medical comorbidities, such as pulmonary disease, coronary artery disease, diabetes, and history of deep venous thrombosis. This did not differ or was a factor among the groups. In fact, the American College of Obstetricians and Gynecologists response is that they support the use of alternatives to hysterectomy, including hormonal management, endometrial ablation, and the use of a levonorgestrel intrauterine device (IUD), as the primary management of these conditions in many cases.[2,5]

Indications for Hysterectomy

There are many reasons or indications for which a hysterectomy should be considered. Some of the indications are displayed below. However, it should be noted that having a problem does not necessarily mean that hysterectomy is the only or best way to treat it. Alternative ways to treat health issues may exist without requiring a hysterectomy. It is important to speak with a gynecologist about all the treatment options available.

Uterine fibroids. Fibroids are benign, non-cancerous tumors or growths made of smooth muscle cells along with fibrous connective tissue that develop within the muscle wall of the uterus and may cause heavy bleeding pain and/or pressure.

Heavy vaginal bleeding. Issues related to hormonal levels, infection, endometrial polyps, cancer, or fibroids can cause heavy, prolonged bleeding.

Uterine prolapse. This is when the uterus lacks support and drops down into the vagina. It is more common in women who had several vaginal births, but it can also happen after menopause or because of obesity. Prolapse can lead to pelvic pressure, along with urinary and bowel problems.

Endometriosis: This chronic and painful disease occurs when the endometrium, the lining of the uterus cavity is displaced outside of the uterus. It can be present on the ovaries, other parts of the pelvis or even distant areas such as the lungs. The endometrial tissue that grows outside of the uterus is called a lesion or an implant. These lesions are fueled by the sex hormone estrogen. When estrogen levels rise, these lesions (patches of endometrial tissue) can grow and later in the menstrual cycle, they may break down and shed. This can even cause pain throughout the month.

Adenomyosis: This is a condition in which the inner lining of the uterus migrates through the myometrium (muscle wall of the uterus). Adenomyosis can cause menstrual cramps, lower abdominal pressure, and heavy periods. The condition can be located throughout the entire uterus or localized in one area.

Cancer or precancer of the uterus, ovary, cervix, or endometrium.
Hysterectomy may be the best option if one has cancer in one of these areas. Other treatment options may include chemotherapy and radiation. An important discussion is necessary with your gynecologist about the type of cancer and the ramification associated with the various treatment options.

How a Hysterectomy is Performed

A hysterectomy can be performed in several ways, depending on one's health history and the reason for the surgery. The type of procedure, risks, possible complications, length of incapacitation along with alternatives to surgery should be discussed with one's gynecologist.

- **Abdominal hysterectomy.** Involves taking out the uterus via an incision in the lower abdomen.
- **Vaginal hysterectomy.** This procedure is performed by taking the uterus out through the vagina via a small incision.
- **Laparoscopic hysterectomy.** Uses a laparoscope, which is an instrument with a thin, lighted cylinder that allows visualization of the pelvic organs. Laparoscopic surgery utilizes a small umbilical incision, followed by insertion of the laparoscope and surgical instruments in the abdomen. During a laparoscopic hysterectomy the uterus is removed through the small incisions made in either the abdomen or vagina.
- **Robotic surgery.** With this procedure a robotic arm is used to perform the surgery through small incisions in the lower abdomen, similar to a laparoscopic hysterectomy. [6]

Possible Hysterectomy Complications and Side Effects

As with any surgery, there are certain complications that may arise with a hysterectomy, including:

- Infection
- Bleeding
- Blood clots in the leg that can travel to the lungs.
- Anesthesia-related complications with the lungs or heart.
- Damage, to surrounding areas, like the bladder, urethra, blood vessels, and nerves
- Bowel obstruction
- Fistula formation (A fistula is an abnormal pathway between two organs, such as the bladder and vagina (called a vesico-vaginal fistula)

A person's medical history may make them more or less prone to developing complications. For instance, people who are obese are more prone to infection and blood clots than those who are at normal weight.

The reason behind the surgery is another risk factor for developing complications. For example, fistula formation (although uncommon) is more likely to occur in people undergoing a hysterectomy for cancer compared to those undergoing a hysterectomy for benign gynecological conditions like pelvic organ prolapse.

The type of hysterectomy a person is undergoing also affects their risk. For example, compared to a vaginal or laparoscopic hysterectomy, an abdominal hysterectomy carries, an increased risk for complications such as infection, bleeding, blood clots, nerve damage, and bowel obstruction.

An abdominal hysterectomy also usually requires the longest hospital stay and recovery time. In contrast, a laparoscopic hysterectomy typically involves a smaller incision, less pain, and a lower risk of infection.

Adverse Effects

There are several potential adverse effects that may occur following a hysterectomy. These are primarily related to physical, emotional, and sexual issues.

Physical adverse effects of undergoing a hysterectomy include postoperative pain, vaginal bleeding, discharge or drainage. Constipation is also common, and some people may experience difficulties with urination or nausea and vomiting. In addition, if the ovaries are removed, people who have not yet entered menopause will no longer menstruate. This is called surgically induced menopause.

As a result, one may experience a range of menopausal symptoms, such as:

- Hot flashes
- Mood swings
- Night sweats
- Vaginal dryness

It's also true that women whose ovaries are not removed, may still experience early menopause. This may be due to compromised blood flow to the ovaries.

Emotional adverse effects may also occur after a hysterectomy. While most people feel satisfied that their symptoms of pelvic pain, vaginal bleeding or other issues are gone, some people in their childbearing years may feel anxious and depressed about the loss of fertility. As such one should communicate and discuss the problem with their gynecologist.

Sexual adverse effects are also a possibility. Fortunately, research shows that most people who were sexually active before surgery, usually experience the same or better sexual functioning after surgery. Sexual functioning after a hysterectomy is really a complicated topic, as every woman is different, and there are many factors to consider, such as:

- Age
- The reason behind having the surgery (cancer versus a non-cancerous condition)
- The level of support provided by a person's partner
- Mood problems that existed before the surgery

A hysterectomy is a common and generally safe surgical procedure, however, as can be expected complications and perhaps unforeseen emotional reactions, do occur.[7,8,9]

Alternatives to Hysterectomies

Hysterectomy is a major surgical procedure and there are many rea-sons for indications for which it should be considered. However, it is important to note that having a health problem does not necessarily mean that a hysterectomy is the only or best way to treat it.

92 | UNNECESSARY HYSTERECTOMIES

Thus, it is crucial to be aware that there may be alternative treatments for one's health issue without resorting to a hysterectomy.

It is essential to carry out thorough research, obtain information through booklets, flyers, and videos about one's specific problem and the various available options. Additionally, it is crucial to have an extensive and informative consultation with one's gynecologist about all treatment options.[10]

Obtaining a second opinion can also be a useful tool, as well as engaging with organizations such as the HERS Foundation (Hysterectomy Resources and Educational Services Foundation) and state and federal agencies, which have a wealth of valuable information.[14]

A few of the treatment options are presented below:

- **Watchful waiting.** Essentially one may wish to wait. This can be applicable for several reasons or cases. However, a common example is in the case of fibroids where menopause is approaching. As such uterine fibroids tend to shrink after menopause. Further the other related adverse problems tend to abate.

- **Exercises.** For uterine prolapse, Kegel exercises (squeezing the pelvic floor muscles) may be beneficial. The exercises have been shown to be helpful in some individuals. By restoring tone to the muscles holding the uterus in place.

- **Medication.** Over-the-counter pain medicines taken during one's period may be helpful. Hormonal birth control, such as the pill, shot, or vaginal ring, or a hormonal intrauterine device (IUD), may help with irregular or heavy vaginal bleeding or periods that last longer than usual. Injectable long-acting gonadotropin-releasing hormone (GnRH) agonists (leuprolide acetate) are effective; however, hypoestrogenic issues limit their duration of use. Another option is the administration of additional hormonal therapy to mitigate side effects. New oral GnRH antagonists (elagolix and relugolix), administered with estradiol and norethindrone acetate, reduce heavy menstrual bleeding, pelvic pain, and anemia in women with uterine fibroids. They are approved for the treatment of uterine fibroids for 24 months. [12,13] Additionally, elagolix alone is currently approved for up to 24 months for the treatment of endometriosis. Furthermore, elagolix and relugolix, when combined with estradiol and norethindrone acetate, are being developed for the treatment of pelvic pain associated with endometriosis. Many gynecologists have reported extraordinary results and exceptional patient satisfaction, with both elagolix and relugolix in the treatment of endometriosis and fibroid tumors symptoms, leading to the opinion that elagolix and relugolix are game changers.[12]

- **Vaginal pessary (for uterine prolapse).** A pessary is a rubber or plastic donut-shaped object, similar to a diaphragm used for birth control. The pessary is inserted into the vagina to hold the uterus in place. Uterine prolapse can occur when the uterus drops or "falls out" because it loses support after childbirth or pelvic surgery.

- **Surgery.** You and your gynecologist may choose to try a surgical procedure that involves smaller or fewer incisions. The smaller incisions may help one to heal faster with less scarring. Depending on one's symptoms, these options may include:

- **Surgery to treat endometriosis.** Laparoscopic surgery uses a thin lighted telescope like instrument which is placed in the abdomen through a small incision. The abdomen is then inflated with C02 gas, which allows the pelvis and abdominal cavity to be viewed on a monitor. Using a small camera attached to one of the instruments, this procedure can remove scar tissue or growths (implants), from endometriosis without harming the surrounding healthy organs such as ovaries. After this surgery you may still be able to get pregnant.

- **Surgery to help stop heavy or extended vaginal bleeding.** Dilation and curettage (D&C) is a procedure that removes the lining of the uterus that builds up every month before the period. Often, a hysteroscopy is done at the same time. The procedure involves insertion of the hysteroscope (a thin telescope) into the uterus to see the inside of the uterine cavity. D&C may also remove noncancerous growths or polyps from the uterus. After the D&C, a new uterine lining will build up during the next menstrual cycle as usual. You may still get pregnant after this surgery. Endometrial ablation destroys the lining of the uterus permanently. Depending on the size and condition of the uterus, ablation may involve use of tools that freeze, heat, or use microwave energy to destroy the uterine lining. This procedure should not be used if you still desire to become pregnant.

- **Surgery to remove uterine fibroids without removing the uterus.** This is called a myomectomy. Depending on the size and location of the fibroids, a myomectomy can be done via laparoscopy, robotic surgery, or abdominal laparotomy. It can also be done through the pelvic area or through the vagina and cervix. One may still be able to get pregnant after this surgery. [14, 15]

o **Surgery to shrink fibroids without removing the uterus.** This is called myolysis. The surgeon treats the fibroids by utilizing a laser or by freezing them, causing them to shrink and degenerate. Myolysis may be done laparoscopically (through very small cuts in the abdominal area). One may still get pregnant after myolysis.

o **Treatments to shrink fibroids.** These treatments include uterine artery embolization (UAE) and magnetic resonance (MR)-guided focused ultrasound (MR[f]US). UAE involves putting tiny plastic or gel particles into the vessels supplying blood to the fibroid. Once the blood supply is blocked, the fibroid shrinks and degenerates. MR(f)US sends ultrasound waves to the fibroids that heat and shrink them. After UAE or MR(f)US, one may not be able to get pregnant. [16, 17]

Take Away

There are always options, make sure you get them from your gynecologist or via a second opinion.

SECTION IV

DIAGNOSIS AND TREATMENT

CHAPTER XI
How Endometriosis is Diagnosed

Endometriosis is one of the most underdiagnosed, misdiagnosed, and mistreated diseases in women of reproductive age. On average, it takes 4-11 years for a patient to receive a diagnosis of endometriosis. The primary cause of this diagnostic delay is the normalization of symptoms by both healthcare professionals and patients. This can have a profound impact on women's lives, including pain, infertility, and decreased quality of life, as well as interference with daily activities, relationships, and livelihood. [4,5]

Clearly, the first step in alleviating or abating these adverse outcomes is to diagnose the underlying condition. For many women, the journey to endometriosis diagnosis is long and arduous with multiple barriers and misdiagnoses. Some of the challenges include a gold standard based on a surgical procedure (laparoscopy), diverse symptomatology contributing to the well-established delay from first symptom onset to surgical diagnosis. It's important to note that remedying the diagnostic delay requires increased patient

100 | How Endometriosis is Diagnosed

education, timely referral to a gynecologist and a shift in the gynecological approach to the disorder. [6]

Endometriosis should be approached as a chronic, systemic, inflammatory, and wide-ranging disease that presents mainly with symptoms of pelvic pain and/or infertility. Therefore, rather than focusing primarily on surgical findings such as implants and adhesions, a clinical approach may be more advantageous. Using this approach, symptoms, signs, and clinical findings of endometriosis would likely become the main drivers of clinical diagnosis and earlier intervention. [7] Combining these factors into a practical guide is expected to simplify endometriosis diagnosis and make the process accessible to more clinicians and patients, which will in essence lead to earlier effective treatment and management.

Embracing the clinical diagnostic paradigm, as proposed by an *Algorithm for a Clinical Diagnosis of Endometriosis*, *(see table 10)*, would involve modifying the following conventional approach to diagnosing endometriosis: *"The history suggests endometriosis, pelvic examination corroborates it, and direct visualization or biopsy verifies it. The definitive diagnosis of endometriosis can only be made by direct observation of endometriosis implants at laparoscopy or laparotomy."*[7,8] (See table 11)

Table 10: Algorithm for a Clinical Diagnosis of Endometriosis [7]
Consistent with Endometriosis

Evaluation Presence of Symptoms	Perform Physical Examination
• Consistent and/or constant pelvic pain	• Nodules in the cul de sac obvious
• Dysmenorrhea	• Retroverted uterus
• Deep Dyspareunia (painful intercourse)	• Mass consistent with endometriosis
• Dyschezia (painful defecation)	• Obvious endometrioma that is external (seen via speculum exam or on the skin)
• Cyclic menstrual symptoms located in other systems such as lungs, skin etc.	
Review Patient History	**Perform/Order Imaging**
• Infertility	• Endometrioma on ultrasound
• Dysmenorrhea in adolescence, current chronic pain	• Pelvic nodules and masses
• Dysmenorrhea unresponsive to anti-inflammatory drugs	
• Positive family history	

102 | HOW ENDOMETRIOSIS IS DIAGNOSED

Clearly the time has come to minimize delays in endometriosis diagnosis and treatment, which would benefit women worldwide. Furthermore, endometriosis has such wide-ranging and pervasive impact that it has been described as "nothing short of a public health emergency," requiring immediate action.[1] Population-based data suggest that more than 4 million reproductive-age women have been diagnosed with endometriosis in the United States. As consequential as this number is it's only part of the story, as an estimated 6 of 10 endometriosis cases are undiagnosed. Thus, more than 6 million American women may experience the effects of endometriosis without understanding the cause of their symptoms or receiving appropriate management. [9]

Pelvic pain and infertility are the two most common endometriosis symptoms. However, the real cost is even greater: women with endometriosis experience diminished quality of life, along with increased incidence of depression and adverse effects on intimate relationships. They also face limitations relevant to participation in daily activities, reduced social activity, loss of productivity and associated income, and increased risk of chronic disease. In addition, there are significant direct and indirect healthcare costs. Furthermore, emerging data indicates that endometriosis is associated with a greater risk of obstetrical and neonatal complications. [10]

Medical History

A thorough history is extremely important, as it acts as a guide to ascertain the name of the pain or other symptoms relevant to endometriosis. Items such as menarche (the first menstrual period) before 11 years old, is associated with a risk for endometriosis.[11]

Relevant to medical illnesses, endometriosis is associated with various disorders such as hypothyroidism, fibromyalgia, chronic fatigue syndrome, autoimmune diseases, allergies, and asthma. Additionally, they are all significantly more common in women with endometriosis than in women in the general population of the United States.[12] Another important factor is that a family history of endometriosis increases the risk of developing endometriosis in fact, it's 7 to 10 times higher than those with no family history. [13] Women with low parity, heavy menses, short menstrual cycles less than 27 days and long duration of menstrual flow are also at increased risk of endometriosis. Furthermore, environmental toxins may increase the risk of endometriosis as stated in the chapter on endometriosis and environmental toxins. Lastly regarding the history, it is also of import to discern the location, frequency, and intensity of pain. [13]

Risk factors for endometriosis include the following: [14, 15, 16]

- Early age of menarche.
- Short menstrual cycles (< 27 d).
- Long duration of menstrual flow (>7 d).
- Heavy bleeding during menses.
- Medical disorders, such as fibromyalgia, hypothyroidism, autoimmune diseases, lupus, etc.
- Inverse relationship to parity (the number of children borne by a woman).
- Delayed childbearing.
- Family history of endometriosis.
- Residing in an environmental toxin challenged area.

Physical Examination

Physical examination is important to help confirm clinical suspicion. Physical exam findings in patients with endometriosis vary and depend to a large extent on the location and stage of the disease. The abdominal examination may note tenderness, particularly in the area where the cyclic pain occurs (lower right side, left side or center). The pelvic examination in mild disease may be normal but with more advanced disease, tenderness, nodularity of the posterior cul de sac and uterosacral ligaments may be appreciated, as well as fixed tender retroversion of the uterus and thickening or masses of the rectrovaginal septum. [17] Adnexal involvement is characterized by ovarian discord with or without tenderness. The exam may be complemented with the vaginal ultrasound probe via *Probe Directed Pelvic Pain Assessment* (PDPPA), whereby pelvic tenderness (rated on a scale of 0-4+) can be evaluated in the right adnexa, left adnexa and central pelvis. Speculum examination may reveal lesions on the surface of the cervix or in the vagina. Umbilical (navel) lesions may be visible and tender on palpation. Pain or bleeding from any site coinciding with menses should raise the index of suspicion leading to careful evaluation of the specific anatomic areas such as lungs, inguinal canal, umbilicus, and/or previous surgical incisions.[18]

Imaging

Imaging techniques used for the diagnosis of endometriosis consists of radiography, ultrasonography computed tomography (CT) and magnetic resonance imaging (MRI). In general, these techniques are of limited value in the diagnosis of endometriosis. Ultrasonography is highly accurate for assessing pelvic and adnexal masses as such may be helpful to differentiate between solid and cystic masses and identify their exact location. This information is particularly useful in formulating preoperative decisions regarding a laparoscopic approach versus laparotomy. CT scanning is a more expensive technique that requires radiation exposure and does not offer much additional information related to the diagnosis and management of pelvic tumors. [19] MRI, on the other hand, does not expose the patient to radiation but is very expensive and may not be readily available in all institutions. However, it has been shown to be effective in the detecting rectovaginal endometriosis nodules and deep infiltrating endometriosis of the uterosacral ligaments. Additionally, it is reliable in determining the size and location of ovarian cysts and possibly large endometriomas. However, MRI alone cannot establish a specific diagnosis of endometriosis. Presently it should be reserved for unusual cases and those with diagnostic problems. [19]

Serum Markers

Cancer Antigen-125 (CA 125) is an antigen associated with a high molecular weight glycoprotein that is expressed on several tissues derived from human celomic (body cavity) epithelium. It was originally found to be expressed in many epithelial ovarian cancers. Using this monoclonal antibody, CA-125 may be detected in the serum of patients with ovarian cancer as well as endometriosis, fibroids, pelvic inflammatory disease (PID) and ovarian hyperstimulation syndrome. CA-125 may also be elevated during pregnancy and with diseases such as appendicitis, chronic liver disease and peritonitis. However, CA 125 is not a sensitive test for endometriosis (52%) and therefore it is not helpful in ruling out the disease. Approximately one-half of the women with histologically proven endometriosis

106 | HOW ENDOMETRIOSIS IS DIAGNOSED

have normal CA 125 levels.[20] The concentration of CA-125 does seems to correlate with both the severity and the clinical course of endometriosis. The response of endometriosis to medical or surgical therapy may be monitored by serial determination of CA-125 levels.

Table 11: Conventional Diagnosis of Endometriosis [8]

Gold Standard	Direct visualization of endometriotic lesions via laparoscopy or laparotomy
Signs and Symptoms	Secondary dysmenorrhea - dyspareunia - infertility
Gyn Exam – Imaging	Ultrasound - MRI - CT - etc.

Laparoscopy

Diagnostic laparoscopy is the "gold standard," for the diagnosis of endometriosis. The minimally invasive surgical procedure is generally performed as an outpatient and requires general anesthesia. A panoramic view of the pelvis can be appreciated with the insertion of a laparoscope (with the use of an attached camera and video monitors) into the abdominal cavity. This is done via a single small umbilical incision, or with an additional suprapubic incision. Robotic laparoscopy can also be utilized which generally requires more than two incisions. No other currently available examination comes close to the diagnostic accuracy of laparoscopy. [21] Additionally, biopsies of endometriotic lesions can be obtained during the procedure to help establish the diagnosis. The typical endometriosis lesions can appear as clear blebs, superficial "powder-burn" or "gunshot" lesion and may black, dark-brown, or blue. Subtle lesions may also be present, which are red or clear and peritoneal defects, small cysts with hemorrhage, and white areas of fibrosis which may also indicate endometriosis.

Fortunately, the patency of the fallopian can be examined by the passage of dye through the reproductive tract. This is of particular importance for infertility patients. The utility of laparoscopy enables the surgeon to employ *"the principle of see and treat,"* by excising any visible endometriosis lesions during the same operation.

Furthermore, at the completion of laparoscopy, it is important to carefully document the extent and stage of endometriosis. The revised scoring system of the American Society for Reproductive Medicine is used to determine the disease stage which ranges from I, (indicating minimal disease) to IV, (indicating severe disease).

This is based on the type, location, appearance, and depth of invasion of the lesions, along with the extent of disease and adhesions. Although staging is useful in determining disease burden and management, the stage does not correlate with the severity of pain, nor does it predict the response to therapies for pain or infertility. Only in this way can the severity of endometriosis be properly assessed, and its course monitored.

For many women the long interval or delay between symptom onset and diagnosis results in prolonged pain decreased quality of life, psychological stress, and impaired fertility. The complex diagnostic challenge of endometriosis is a quadruple of nonspecific symptoms, a lack of sensitive and specific biomarkers and a lack of awareness on the part of both the public, and healthcare professionals.

More specifically, the challenge is variable with symptoms such as dysmenorrhea, dyspareunia, dyschezia, and infertility, which can be attributed to many conditions. In addition, these symptoms are often not discussed openly because of the fear of being disparaged. Furthermore, awareness of the disease is poor on the part of the general public, employers, and persons in health care professions. As a result of these factors, the average delay between the onset of symptoms and diagnosis is 4-11 years. To remedy this, it is important to increase patient education, healthcare professionals' education, timely referral to an endometriosis specialist and enhance funding for endometriosis research.

Take Away

- It's important to listen to one's body and trust your instincts. If you think you might have endometriosis, it's worth it to seek out an endometriosis specialist.
- Knowing the risk factors for endometriosis can help to manage one's health. Not only does this information supply effective risk reduction strategies. It can also help one's endometriosis specialist arrive at a more accurate diagnosis.
- Since endometriosis is easily misdiagnosed, identifying the risk factors for this condition can narrow down the search for the cause of one's symptoms.
- With a diagnosis comes solutions, so it's imperative to discuss the risk factors for endometriosis with an endometriosis specialist.

CHAPTER XII
HOW ENDOMETRIOSIS IS TREATED

The treatment of endometriosis depends on its clinical manifestations which currently fall into two categories: pelvic pain and/or infertility. The treatment for endometriosis can involve one or a combination of medical treatments. It could be conservative or definitive surgery, or a combination of medical and surgical treatments.[1,2] Expectant management is generally reserved for patients without significant symptoms and for those approaching menopause. However even those with few symptoms benefit from treatment aimed at preventing progression of the disease. Endometriosis normally regresses after menopause due to the marked decrease in ovarian estrogen production. As such perimenopausal women with mild symptoms may choose expectant management or treatment limited to nonnarcotic analgesics for the short term.[3] Young women with significant symptoms generally will require more aggressive medical or surgical treatment.

110 | How Endometriosis is Treated

Currently, the treatment choices for symptomatic endometriosis are determined by the patient's preferences, treatment goals, the side-effect profile, efficacy, costs, associated comorbidities, and availability.[4]

Medical Treatment

Empirical medical therapy is commonly initiated for pain control without surgical confirmation of disease. Such therapy is intended to reduce pain through a variety of mechanisms which include minimizing inflammation, interrupting, or suppressing cyclic ovarian hormone production, inhibiting the action and synthesis of estradiol and reducing or eliminating menses.[4]

Women with pelvic pain, suspected endometriosis, and no other indication for surgical treatment can be managed effectively with empiric medical treatment without establishing a surgical diagnosis. Initial empiric medical therapy usually involves treatment with NSAIDs and oral contraceptives (OCPs: combined or progestin only). If treatment with NSAIDs and OCPs does not significantly improve pain, then second and third-line medical therapies or laparoscopic surgery should be considered.[5]

Traditionally medical therapies for endometriosis have been to reduce or eliminate cyclic menstruation. This reduces peritoneal seeding and the likelihood that new implants developing. These therapies also aim to suppress the growth and activity of the endometrium in anticipation of the same occurring in endometriotic tissue derived from it. Interventions that reduce ovarian estradiol production are the most reliable ways to cause atrophy of endometriotic lesions and the most effective treatment for pain. These concepts have shaped medical treatment for endometriosis for years.

However, our growing understanding of the molecular pathogenesis of endometriosis is now beginning to suggest new treatment strategies aimed at the mechanisms of disease. [4,6]

Nonsteroidal Anti-inflammatory Medications

Nonsteroidal anti-inflammatory medications (NSAIDs) are the widely used first-line medication for primary dysmenorrhea or pain associated with endometriosis. Additionally, they have an added desired anti-inflammatory effect and are typically used in conjunction with oral contraceptives. [7]

Estrogen–Progestin Contraceptives

Estrogen-progestin contraceptives have been the mainstay of the medical treatment of symptomatic endometriosis. They are the most prescribed treatment and are well-tolerated by most women. Continuous treatment can eliminate menses and is the preferred method for those with dysmenorrhea. The most frequently encountered problem is unscheduled "breakthrough" bleeding or spotting, which usually becomes less frequent the longer one takes the medication. Estrogen-progestin contraceptives can be expected to provide effective relief from pain associated with endometriosis in up to two-thirds of affected women, particularly when taken continuously. [8,9,10]

Progestins

Progestins have long been used to treat symptomatic endometriosis. They inhibit endometrial growth and presumably the growth of endometriotic tissue. Initially, they induce decidualization and then

112 | HOW ENDOMETRIOSIS IS TREATED

atrophy occurs. In high doses they can inhibit ovulation and initiate amenorrhea.

Continuous Progestin Hormonal Therapy

Progestins, are one of the components found in combined estrogen/progestin treatments, like the birth control pill (see medical treatments: continuous estrogen/progestin). Progestins alone are also effective in treating endometriosis, particularly when taken in a long-term continuous fashion. Furthermore, progestins tend to thin the lining of the uterus, which stops regular periods and lessens the chance for break-through bleeding or spotting.[11]

Gonadotropin–Releasing Hormone Analogues

GnRH Agonists. GnRH agonists are analogs of the hormone GnRH. This hypothalamic hormone is responsible for stimulating the pituitary gland to secrete follicle-stimulating hormone (FSH) and luteinizing hormone (LH), which are necessary for normal ovarian function. GnRH agonists induce down-regulation of the pituitary-ovarian axis, leading to hypoestrogenism, amenorrhea and endometrial atrophy. However, GnRH agonist induce menopausal symptoms, such as hot flushes, vaginal dryness, decreased libido, mood swings, headaches, and bone mineral depletion. GnRH agonist can be delivered via a nasal spray or subcutaneous injections.

Gonadotropin-releasing hormone (GnRH) agonists substantially suppress systemic estrogen levels. The menopause-like side effects, including bone loss, can be decreased by adding low-dose estrogen replacement therapy [12]

GnRH Antagonist. GnRH antagonists are relatively new oral non-peptides that are available for the treatment of endometriosis-associated pain. The oral GnRH antagonists produce a dose dependent hypoestrogenic environment by direct pituitary gonadotropin suppression which inhibits endometriotic cell proliferation and invasion, while maintaining sufficient circulating estradiol levels to avoid vasomotor symptoms, vaginal atrophy, and bone demineralization. Unlike GnRH agonists, antagonists do not stimulate the receptor and therefore there is no flare effect (increase in symptoms). They directly block the GnRH receptor and can function rapidly with a partial dose-dependent reduction in gonadotropins. Given their rapid onset oral administration, absence of flare effect and the availability of tailoring therapy, they may be considered the first choice for patients not responding to OCPs or those with side effects from progestins. It should be noted that complete suppression of ovulation does not occur; thus, concomitant contraception is needed in women who are at risk for pregnancy.[13, 14]

Danazol. Danazol is an androgen and one of the first drugs ever approved for the treatment of endometriosis in the United States in the 1970s. It inhibits steroidogenesis and the LH surge, thereby increasing free testosterone levels. Due to the increase in androgen levels, potential side effects include hirsutism, acne and deepening of the voice. Danazol has proven effective for reducing endometriosis related pain (dysmenorrhea, deep dyspareunia, intermenstrual pain) in up to 90% of treated women. However, it is rarely used now because of its substantial androgenic and hypoestrogenic side effects. [11]

114 | HOW ENDOMETRIOSIS IS TREATED

Aromatase Inhibitors. Aromatase inhibitors (AIs), aromatase is an enzyme that converts steroidal precursors into estrogen causing ectopic tissue to grow and leading to the onset of pelvic pain. Inhibition of aromatase reduces estrogen levels causing atrophy of endometriotic lesions and is one of the most effective treatments of endometriosis.

Aromatase inhibitors are associated with hot flashes, mild headache, nausea, myalgia, and in premenopausal women, ovarian cyst formation. Most studies evaluating the use of aromatase inhibitors combine them with oral contraceptives or norethindrone acetate (NETA) to avoid the follicular engagement, ovarian stimulation, and ovarian cyst formation associated with the elevated follicle-stimulating hormone levels induced by aromatase inhibitor activity.[4,11]

Future Therapeutics

Recent studies have focused on the potential benefits of selective progesterone receptor modulators (SPRMs) in the managing of endometriosis-associated pain. Mifepristone was found to decrease pain symptoms and induce amenorrhea in endometriosis patients. Other agents such as statins, COX-2 inhibitors and dopamine agonists are currently being evaluated. However clinical evidence is not yet available to support their effectiveness.[15] Additionally intracrinology which is the study of hormones that act inside a cell, is being used to address diseases through a new tissue-specific approach. [16, 17]

ENDOMETRIOSIS | 115

Table 12: Current Hormone Medication Options to Treat Pelvic pain Associated with Endometriosis [18]

Medication	Elago-lix	Relugolix	Leupro-lide	Medroxy -proges-terone	Letrozole	Danazol
Class /Mechanism of Action	GnRH Antagonist	GnRH Antagonist	GnRH Agonist	Progestin	Aromatase Inhibitor	Androgen
Route of Administration	Oral	Oral	IM	SC	Oral	Oral
Dose	150 mg daily or 200 mg twice daily for 6-24 months	relugolix 40mg/ estradiol 1mg/ norethindrone 0.5mg, daily for up to 24 months	3.75 mg monthly (6 months add back 12 months)	104 mg Every 3 months up to 24 months	2.5 mg daily with norethindrone	200-800 mg twice daily
Contraindication	√	√	√	√	√	√
Bone Loss	√	√	√	√	√	
Menstrual Bleeding Pattern	√	√	√			
Treatment Options	√	√			√	√
Adverse Reactions	√	√	√	√	√	
Race & Weight			√			

116 | HOW ENDOMETRIOSIS IS TREATED

Table 13: Endometriosis should be viewed as a chronic condition that requires a lifelong management plan [19,20]

Initial Medical Management	Other Medical Management	Surgical Management
NSAIDs (OTC and prescription)	Progestin (subcutaneously or via an IUD	Laparoscopy or Laparotomy
Combined hormonal contraception (cyclic or continuous)	GnRH agonists GnRH antagonist	Neurectomy
Progestin (oral)	Androgen (Danazol)	Hysterectomy and oophorectomy

Surgical Treatment

The objectives or aim of surgical treatment for endometriosis is to excise or destroy all visible endometriotic tissue and adhesions to the extent possible and to restore normal anatomical relationships to prevent or delay recurrence. However, success in achieving this aim may largely depend on the skill of the surgeon. Additionally, women with moderate or severe endometriosis that distorts the reproductive anatomy hope to restore or preserve fertility. Medical treatment cannot achieve this goal, and surgery is the treatment of choice. When the disease is less severe, medical treatment may effectively control pain in most women. However, it offers little or no effect on fertility. Surgery is at least as effective as medical treatment for relieving pain and may improve fertility.[7,21]

Surgery for the treatment of endometriosis can be performed via laparoscopy (straight/robotic) or laparotomy. Recent technical advances in instrumentation and technique generally allow for the laparoscopy approach. In all but those who require extensive surgery and even that can be performed by highly skilled surgeons via laparoscopy. Laparoscopy also offers the advantage of better visualization, less tissue trauma, smaller incisions, and a speedier postoperative recovery. Additionally, the results achieved with laparoscopy are equivalent to or better than with laparotomy. [22]

Regardless of the surgical approach, a system of classification or staging of endometriosis is useful to better describe the extent of disease, develop meaningful diagnostic modalities and treatments, as well as to enhance research and standardize communication between health professionals. [3]

Endometriosis presents in many different forms, with a wide variety of clinical presentations. Therefore, a unified consensus classification system for the stage of the disease is not a simple task. The most widely used and best-known worldwide was developed by the American Society for Reproductive Medicine (ASRM). The Revised ASRM (rASRM) classification system is divided into four stages according to the number of lesions and depth of infiltration: minimal (Stage I), mild (Stage II), moderate (Stage III), and severe (Stage IV). It is very easy for health professionals to apply and for patients to understand. However, it has some limitations such as a poor correlation between the extent of disease expressed by rASRM score and pain symptoms, infertility, or patient quality of life. Regarding prognosis, there is no correlation with infertility outcome and only poor predictive accuracy of treatment outcome. [23, 24]

118 | HOW ENDOMETRIOSIS IS TREATED

Table 14: ASRM Endometriosis Stages: [23, 24]

Endometriosis Stage	Manifestation of the Condition
Stage I (1-5 points)	Minimal Few superficial implants
Stage II (6-15 points)	Mild More and deeper implants
Stage III (16-40 points)	Moderate Many deep implants Small cysts on one or both ovaries
Stage IV (>40 points)	Severe Many deep implants Large cysts on one or both ovaries Many dense adhesions

This points system has its limitations and doesn't always accurately match the patients' symptoms or likelihood to get pregnant.

Relevant to **minimal and mild disease**, endometriotic peritoneal implants may be ablated with electrosurgical instruments or laser or excised by sharp dissection. Adhesions associated with endometriosis that distort the reproductive anatomy should be excised even though adhesion reformation may reoccur. "Excision is preferable to simple lysis because adhesions frequently contain disease. Of course, strict adherence to the use of methods that embrace minimum tissue trauma and meticulous hemostasis is necessary." [25, 26]

Moderate and severe disease which encompasses ovarian endometriomas and deep infiltrating endometriosis involving the recto-vaginal septum requires extensive surgery. Regarding endometriomas, surgical technique is important because excision of excessive tissue or significant damage can compromise ovarian function. [25,26]

In women with advance symptomatic endometriosis who have completed childbearing, as well as those in whom medical and conservative surgical treatment fails, definitive surgical treatment or hysterectomy deserves serious consideration. In highly selected women having no significant ovarian disease, hysterectomy alone can be considered. However, the risk of recurrent disease requiring additional treatment is approximately 6-fold higher, especially, when oophorectomy (removal of ovaries) is not performed. Other risk factors for persistent or recurrent endometriosis and pain include incomplete excision of disease and postoperative estrogen therapy in women with extensive or residual disease. However, when all visible endometriosis is removed, the risk for recurrent pain in women who receive immediate or delayed hormone treatment is similar.[27]

Key Points

- Established medical therapies for the treatment of pain associated with endometriosis include estrogen-progestin contraceptives, progestins, GnRH analogs and danazol.
- Treatment decisions should be individualized after carefully considering the severity of symptoms, the extent of disease, the desire for future pregnancy, age, side-effects, and costs.
- Relevant to classification systems for endometriosis the ASRM revised classification is the most widely used.
- Research is ongoing for the development of new therapeutic agents.

Take Away

- Endometriosis should be viewed as a chronic disease that requires a lifelong management plan.
- If treatment with NSAIDs and OCPs does not significantly improve pain; second and third-line medical therapies or laparoscopic surgery should be considered.
- Definitive treatment of endometriosis with hysterectomy and bilateral salpingoooophorectomy should be reserved for women with debilitating symptoms, that can reasonably be attributed to the disease. These women should have completed childbearing and have failed to respond to alternative treatments.

CHAPTER XIII
ALTERNATIVE WAYS TO REPRESS ENDOMETRIOSIS

Recently, we have been fortunate to have a number of new medications such as elagolix and relugolix added to our armamentarium in the fight against endometriosis.[1,2] However, in terms of treatment, they may not be suitable for everyone. Fortunately, there are a variety of other supportive measures. These measures could range from devising a healthy nutritional plan to relieving pain and stress. Thankfully, there's a multitude of therapies and options that's available, such as acupuncture, massage, physical therapy, diet, and lifestyle modification. Regrettably, none of these supporting therapies take the place of surgery. However, all of them have the capability of helping to improve one's quality of life relevant to endometriosis. It's evident that not every therapy is appropriate for everyone; thus, an individualized treatment plan should be carefully considered. Additionally, for chronic pain a multidisciplinary team approach would be extremely helpful. This should include the gynecologist along with other principals such as physical therapist, psychologist, pain specialist and others.[2]

122 | Alternative Ways to Repress Endometriosis

Acupuncture

Let's look at acupuncture which is an alternative approach to pain management and relaxation. It has been practiced in China for more than 3000 years. It spread throughout Europe and America from the 16th to the 19 centuries. In fact, the history of acupuncture research was initiated in the 18th century and has developed rapidly since then. It has attracted increasing attention as a safe and easy-to-perform treatment. Acupuncture involves placing very thin needles in various strategic places in the body. It is based on the belief that *Chi* or energy flow through pathways (meridians) located in the body and can become blocked or imbalanced, resulting in disease and pain. Placing the needles at specific points along the meridian helps to rebalance this flow. A Western medicine theory is that it may help regulate the nervous system and release pain-suppressing endorphins.[3]

Scientific evidence indicates that acupuncture may be beneficial in helping to reduce the pain associated with endometriosis. As a matter of fact, two recent studies suggest that patients who receive acupuncture treatment tend to be more relaxed. Since muscle tension and stress play an important role in chronic pain symptoms, it is reasonable to note that acupuncture can provide pain relief. Due to such acupuncture should be considered as one of the components of a pain management plan.[4, 5, 6]

Advantageously, acupuncture has evolved from its original methods, to include other methods such as moxibustion (the traditional method of burning the dried leaves of the mugwort plant to stimulate acupuncture points which assist in improving the effect), together with electroacupuncture, auricular(ear), acupoint treatment, and acupuncture combined with other therapies. All of these can effectively relieve the symptoms of pain caused by endometriosis.[5]

Physical Therapy and Massage

Physical therapy and massage can help endometriosis patients successfully manage pain. The goal of these treatments is to decrease stress, improve muscle tone and enhance quality of life for endometriosis patients by helping them relax. Some options to achieve these goals are focused pelvic physical therapy (PT), biofeedback, and transcutaneous electrical nerve (TEN) stimulation. **Biofeedback** teaches patients to alter their response to pain signals, by controlling their heart rate, respirations, muscle tone and temperature. Initially patients learn to recognize and control these responses, by using skin electrodes, which translate physiological changes into auditory or visual signals. **Transcutaneous electrical nerve (TEN) stimulation** is the direct electrical stimulation of the skin overlying pain trigger-points to provide relief. After a complete physical therapy evaluation, patients who may benefit from this treatment can obtain a portable TEN unit to manage their symptoms.[7]

Meditation, Mindfulness, Yoga, Tai Chi, Qigong and Hypnosis

From a positive perspective, improving a person's outlook on life, may help them to cope with problems related to endometriosis. Some mind-body practices involve mindful movement, such as yoga and tai chi. These helps reduce stress and relax muscles, which may decrease pain. Unfortunately, few studies have explored the impact of mind-body practices on endometriosis-related symptoms. Thus, more research needs to be done to better understand this possible link. However, results thus far have shown that mind-body practices may improve a person's overall quality of life. A summary of the listed practices is presented below.[8]

Meditation is a practice that involves focusing the mind. Many forms of meditation involve sitting quietly and alone. Meditation can also occur during prayer. While it is regularly used in some religions, it does not have to be a religious practice. Meditation may also take the form of using guided imagery. Guided imagery relies on the imagination to picture different relaxing situations or locations. The guiding can come from an in-person guide, tapes, or videos. [8]

Mindfulness is often considered a type of meditation. However, it does not always have to take place alone or in one place. Mindfulness can occur at any time or in any place. It involves being aware and present in each moment. During routine events such as driving to work or watching TV, the mind can go on autopilot. However, making an effort to be aware in these moments is a way of practicing mindfulness. Along with taking special care to notice the things going on around you, it is considered practicing mindfulness.[8]

Yoga, tai chi, and qigong are practices that involve tapping into the mind-body connection via physical movement. They are sometimes called mindful movement. They can each take on many forms and intensities, making them accessible to most people. Mindful movement therapies can be performed at a studio or on your own at home with the help of self-guided videos or recordings. [9]

Hypnosis can be performed by a trained professional on a person to induce a trance-like state of deep focus. This focus is generally directed at one thought, idea, task, or object. It causes the person experiencing it to have no other distractions. Hypnosis can also be self-guided in some situations.[9]

Lifestyle Modification

It's reasonable to assume that a positive lifestyle change is likely to have a protective effect, particularly against certain diseases and to achieve wellness. Interestingly, very few studies focused on whether certain diets or levels of activity are connected to endometriosis symptoms or whether these aspects improve endometriosis-related symptoms. On the other hand, exercise, or physical activity appears to have protective effects against diseases that involve inflammatory processes. It induces an increase in the systemic levels of cytokines, which have anti-inflammatory and antioxidant properties, as well as a reduction in estrogen levels.[9]

Exercise and Physical Activities

Evidence has suggested that the symptoms associated with endometriosis result from a local inflammatory peritoneal reaction, which is caused by displaced endometrial implants. It's also known that women who exercise intensely tend to have lighter periods with reduced ovarian stimulation and estrogen production. In one study, researchers evaluated the effects of high-intensity physical activity on a woman's risk of endometriosis. They found that women who averaged 2.5 hours of high-intensity activity (jogging, bicycling or aerobics) per week, were 63 % less likely to have endometriosis. Other studies noted benefits limited to women who exercised more than 4 hours a week.[10]. When exercise is carried out, the brain releases "feel good" chemicals called endorphins. These naturally occurring hormones work like pain relievers to lower pain. Regular exercise also lowers the amount of estrogen in the body. Wherein one of the goals of endometriosis treatment is to lower estrogen levels, which tends to improve endometriosis symptoms. Despite this, it is not possible to ascertain the real role of physical exercise in endometriosis. Intuitively, research is needed to fully answer the question. Thus, if any female diagnosed with endometriosis is wondering? If there is anything that she can do to feel better besides taking medication, clearly exercise may be part of the answer.[10]

Nutrition

Good nutrition is the cornerstone of good health. The proverbial statement, *"you are what you eat,"* is correct: what you put into your body affects how it functions. For women with endometriosis, good nutrition can reduce symptoms and pain and provide a feeling of vitality in their life. Eating well can give you extra energy, help balance your blood sugar, fight insulin resistance, balance your metabolism and control your weight. *Food is medicine when you're dealing with endometriosis.* The basis of a good diet is straightforward: avoid processed foods and eat real foods. Processed foods depletes your energy, while fresh foods, particularly organic ones with plenty of vegetables, help you to feel vivacious. [11]

Not only changing the way you eat but also how much you eat can have a remarkable effect on how you look and feel. *Plainly, excessive amounts of unhealthy food can make you unhealthy,* so always eat in moderation. Foods rich in omega-3 fatty acids with anti-inflammatory effects, in addition to an increased consumption of fruits, vegetable (preferably organic), olive oil and whole grains exert a protective effect. This can reduce the risk of development and possible regression of disease. On the other hand, foods that increase inflammation, such as those that promote the production of pain-producing prostaglandins, are sugar, alcohol, wheat, red meats, and saturated fat.[12] For protein, fish, raw nuts and legumes and small amounts of white meats such as chicken and veal are good choices.[13] In fact every cell of the body requires a building block of protein, which the body uses to repair and heal itself. Lastly don't hesitate to consult a dietician.[14]

Foods That Helps with Endometriosis

Fiber: Excess estrogen is removed by fiber, too much estrogen can aggravate endometriosis symptoms like cramping and pain. Fiber helps to facilitate regular bowel movements which helps to reduce estrogen levels. One can boost fiber by eating more:

- Legumes, like beans, lentil, and chickpea
- Fruits and vegetables
- Whole grains

Inflammation: Endometriosis is an inflammatory condition, thus anti-inflammatory foods like those below may be helpful.

- Fatty fish such as salmon and sardines
- Nuts and seeds, such as almonds, walnuts, chia seeds and flaxseed
- Plant oils such as flaxseed oil, canola oil and olive oil.[15]

Foods to Avoid with Endometriosis

Certain foods may worsen endometriosis pain by boosting inflammation or estrogen levels. One should limit or avoid:

- **Alcohol**: Wine, beer and other spirits may make endometriosis worse. Limit to one or two drinks per week.
- **Caffeine**: Limit the daily caffeine to 400 milligrams or less. One cup of coffee can have over 100 milligrams, depending on how it's brewed.
- **Fatty meat**: Some red meat is good, however limit the overall saturated fat intake to 10% of your daily calories.
- **Processed foods**: Many packaged foods contain pro-inflammatory ingredients like added sugar, saturated fat, and trans-fat.
- **Sugary drinks** (liquid candy bars): Fruit juices, sodas and energy drinks are often high in sugar which can make inflammation worse. Aim for less than 26 grams of sugar daily. [16, 17]

Herbs and Supplements

The following herbs and supplements have been shown, in small to moderate-sized studies to improve the quality of life for those with endometriosis by reducing chronic pain and other related symptoms. They have also been noted to cause regression of endometrial lesions and endometriosis-related ovarian cysts, as well as improve fertility, reduce the need for surgery and improve sleep. Some extracts from herbs and supplements have also been shown to cause regression of endometriosis lesions. Herbal remedies are considered an alternative treatment for endometriosis, and they should be used to support primary treatment under the guidance of a gynecologist. [18,19]

Curcumin

Curcumin is an active ingredient in turmeric and has been shown to have anti-endometriotic effects, which may relieve symptoms of endometriosis. The positive effects are likely due to a combination of its anti-inflammatory and antioxidant properties, along with its ability to increase glutathione, and regulate the immune system, while addressing some of the core immune dysfunctions contributing to endometriosis. [18, 19]

Pycnogenol (Maritime Pine Bark)

Pycnogenol or Pine Bark extract has been known to have many analgesic properties. This extract taken in capsule form has been shown to reduce pain in many conditions from osteoarthritis to dysmenorrhea, which is a common symptom of endometriosis.

This natural supplement has been proven in studies to have lasting and compounding effects. In one study pycnogenol was found to be more effective in treating painful periods in endometriosis than gonadotropin-releasing hormone agonist, a common hormone therapy treatment for endometriosis. Not only were the effects of pycnogenol long lasting, but the results lasted even after discontinuing use. In fact, the longer the supplement was taken, the better results patients received.

Another study showed that the use of pycnogenol significantly reduced pain scores of dysmenorrhea, as well as the need for analgesics. This effect persisted even after the women stopped using the pycnogenol and fewer analgesics were needed. Add to these benefits the fact that pycnogenol has antioxidant properties, and it becomes clear that this supplement may be a valuable addition to the treatment of endometriosis.[18,19]

Melatonin

Melatonin is usually considered as a sleep supplement and is the natural substance that increases at night in our brains to tell us to get some sleep! However, melatonin appears to have quadruple actions with antioxidant, anti-inflammatory, immunoregulatory, and pain-relieving benefits, particularly in the treatment of endometriosis. Melatonin is also a powerful natural detoxifier, especially of excess or harmful forms of estrogen, which may explain its powerful role in endometriosis care.

In one study of 40 women with chronic pelvic pain, who were between 18 and 45 years old, 10 mg of **melatonin** per day was able to significantly:

- Reduce chronic pelvic pain due to endometriosis.
- Reduce pelvic pain during menses and during sex.
- Led to an overall 80% reduction in the need for pain medication in women taking the melatonin, including reduction in NSAIDS and opioid use.

Women in the melatonin group also reported substantially improved sleep and a greater sense of wellness on morning waking. In animal studies, melatonin led to regression and shrinkage of endometriosis tissue. [18, 19]

Ginger

Ginger is a potent anti-inflammatory and powerful antioxidant agent. It contains gingerols which inhibits the formation of inflammatory cytokines, chemical messengers of the immune system. As a result, gingerols have been found to reduce pain when consumed regularly. There has even been a study that found supplementing with ginger to be as effective as ibuprofen and mefenamic acid at reducing painful periods.

Conditions such as endometriosis encourage inflammation in the body. Inflammation produces free radicals, which are waste products produced by cells. If the body doesn't remove free radicals effectively, oxidative stress can occur. Oxidative stress can damage our cells and DNA and can result in disease down the line. So, it's incredibly important that we consume antioxidants in our diet, to combat free radicals and minimize the effects of oxidative stress.

Another symptom associated with endometriosis is nausea during the menstrual phase. Both ginger root powder and fresh ginger have been shown to reduce nausea. [18,19]

N-acetyl-cysteine (NAC)

NAC is a powerful supplement that increases glutathione, one of the most important detoxifiers naturally produced in our bodies. However, many of us aren't producing quite enough, to keep up with the demands put on our bodies by chronic exposure to environmental toxins, in conjunction with the overproduction of our own natural hormones – including estrogen. NAC has some impressive data specifically for endometriosis. In a 2013 study of 92 women in Italy, 47 took NAC and 42 took a placebo. Of those who took 600 mg of NAC three times a day, three consecutive days each week for three months:

- 24 patients cancelled their scheduled laparoscopy due to a decrease or disappearance of endometriosis symptoms, improved pain reduction or because they had gotten pregnant!
- 14 of the women in the NAC group had decreased ovarian cysts.
- 8 had a complete disappearance of their symptoms – and lesions.
- 21 had pain reduction.

In the other group, only 1 patient cancelled surgery. A total of 8 women got pregnant in the NAC group, while 6 did in the placebo-only group. [19]

Green Tea

Epigallocatechin gallate (EGCG), is one of the main polyphenols catechins found in green tea and has antioxidant, anti-angiogenetic and anti-proliferative effects in endometriotic tissue. Many studies aim to prove the various beneficial effects of green tea on human health. Researchers from China and Hong Kong have even written a review, on different molecular and cellular mechanisms of the contents of green tea that prohibit inflammation, oxidative stress, invasion and angiogenesis. They have also explored its potential use, particularly in treating endometriosis.[20,21]

Resveratrol

Resveratrol is a naturally occurring plant-based compound that has anti-inflammatory, anti-estrogenic, antioxidant effects and anti-angiogenic effects. Angiogenesis or blood vessel formation is another essential mechanism, for the creation and subsequent maintenance of lesions found in those with endometriosis. Resveratrol suppresses these angiogenic factors and has been shown to reduce the size and number of lesions. Thus, it is evident that Resveratrol can counteract many of the theorized molecular mechanisms that cause endometriosis. It is abundant in nature and can be found in many different plant species, fungi, berries, peanuts, legumes, and grasses. However, grapes and red wines are considered the primary source of Resveratrol. While Resveratrol does not appear to have an adverse health effect, further testing is required to determine its feasibility as a treatment option. [22,23]

Vitamin B6

Vitamin B6 or pyridoxine is thought to play a role in hormone regulation. It is specifically needed for glutathione production. As such it has been shown to improve hormone related symptoms, such as the intensity and duration of the period pain by reducing the level of estrogen in the body. Although B6 may relieve endometriosis symptoms, more research is needed to better understand the possible link. [18, 24]

134 | ALTERNATIVE WAYS TO REPRESS ENDOMETRIOSIS

Ultimately under the guidance of a patient's primary gynecologist. Some of the often-debilitating symptoms of endometriosis may be successfully alleviated. In addition, it may be advantageous to include a multidisciplinary healthcare team that incorporates alternative therapies.

Take Away

"If endometriosis is interfering with your life, try exercising and changing your diet."

CHAPTER XIV
ADOLESCENTS AND ENDOMETRIOSIS

In the United States it is estimated that more than 6.5 million women and girls as young as eight suffer from endometriosis and more than 190 million worldwide. We know the disease can continue to cause symptoms well into mid-life, and even later. Various studies have indicated that 38% of those with endometriosis have symptoms before the age of 15. Additionally, it takes 4-11 years to receive a correct diagnosis and treatment. This in essence means that much of a child's youth may be spent suffering due to unexplained, often crippling *pain without a name*, which may greatly impede her development.[1,2]

The youngest victims of endometriosis are often the most affected. This is, in part, relevant to the common belief that endometriosis does not affect this age group. It is also because they are often too uncomfortable or perplexed to talk about their symptoms. Frequently, girls with endometriosis discontinue normal activities, miss school, or even drop out. As a result of their pain, which impacts

136 | ADOLESCENTS AND ENDOMETRIOSIS

their academic lives, their future, their families, and their communities. [1,2]

Severe Painful Periods During Adolescence Isn't Normal

Severe painful periods or *killer cramps* are never normal, particularly during adolescence. Some research shows that up to two-thirds of women who suffer from endometriosis had symptoms before they were 20 years old. Explicitly girls who begin experiencing acutely painful periods may have already developed endometriosis. Moreover, severe painful periods are common in adolescence. In fact, an Australian study noted that of 1000 schoolgirls aged 16-18 found that 93% had painful periods. Of these, 21% had severe painful periods and 26% missed school for painful periods or a mixture of menstrual symptoms. [3,4]

Families and physicians should never believe that a girl's severe pain is exaggerated or normal, particularly if the pain is severe enough to keep her away from school or to prevent her from participating in sports and day-to-day activities. When faced with these monumental problems, it's time to find a gynecologist who understands endometriosis along with other causes of pelvic pain in adolescents to assist in receiving the help she deserves. It is particularly important to seek out a specialist early on. This is advisable to ensure that the girls are not traumatized by having their symptoms invalidated and undergoing numerous painful medical tests, taking ineffective medications with severe side effects, as well as to make sure they get relief from their suffering. If it is not endometriosis, the pain is still serious and needs to be evaluated. [2,4]

Risk factors

There are many risk factors associated with endometriosis in adolescents, including genetic, anatomic, and hormonal factors. Endometriosis tends to run in families, so young women with relatives with endometriosis (mothers, sisters, and aunts) have a higher chance of having endometriosis. There is a genetic link to endometriosis in adolescents, as seen with adult patients. In fact, a recent study found a positive family history in a third of cases, while a first-degree relative was affected in a quarter of cases of adolescents with surgically confirmed endometriosis. [5]

Obstructive reproductive tract abnormalities (Mullerian anomalies) can lead to increased retrograde or backward menstruation, which has been shown to increase the risk for endometriosis in adolescents. This is supported by spontaneous improvement of endometriosis symptoms after the obstruction is surgically corrected.

An early age of the first menstrual period or menarche is associated with higher risk of endometriosis. This is thought to be due to increased exposure to estrogen and prolonged duration of retrograde menstruation. Early onset of severe cramps and chronic pelvic pain at the time of menarche, has been shown to increase the probability of having endometriosis. Additionally, a low BMI has also been shown to be correlated with increased risk of endometriosis. [2,3]

Symptoms

In adolescents, the symptoms of endometriosis are generally chronic pelvic pain, while symptoms in adult women are cyclical chronic pelvic pain and progressive worsening dysmenorrhea, as well as dyspareunia in cases where they are sexually active. A more comprehensive list of symptoms is displayed in table 15. Additionally, the localization of endometriosis in the ovary (ovarian endometrioma) is rare before 25 years. Some authors report that diagnostic laparoscopy is necessary for adolescents who experience acyclic chronic pelvic pain and do not respond to oral contraceptives (OCP) and NSAIDS.[6,7]

Table 15: Common Symptoms[7]

Adolescents with endometriosis may experience one or more of the following:

Heavy periods	Pelvic muscle spasm
Bloating	An irritable bowel
Diarrhea	A painful overactive bladder
Nausea	Headaches
Lower back pain	Fatigue
Leg pain	Chronic pain throughout the cycle

Diagnosis

There are a variety of methods that can be used to assess whether a woman has endometriosis, but the only reliable way to confirm the disease is by visually inspecting the pelvic and abdominal areas through laparoscopy or laparotomy. Due to this most women with chronic pelvic pain prefer empirical treatment before considering surgery. Additionally, the recent clinical diagnosis of endometriosis methodology has been helpful in diagnosing endometriosis. Moreover, thanks to modern imaging techniques such as ultrasound and MRI, it is now possible to make a less invasive diagnosis of endometriosis. However, laparoscopy remains the gold standard and most consequential. The diagnostic procedure does not differ in adolescents or adults. However, a careful history is crucial in young women to determinate the chronicity of the pain, related bowel or bladder problems, and responsiveness to medication. Some investigators have suggested a pain or symptom diary (see the *symptom tracker* in the appendix), which allows the patient to describe and document the frequency and character of her symptoms.[8] Adequate family history is also essential information, as the incidence of endometriosis in patients with affected family members is 6.9% compared to 1%-2% for the general population.[8,9]

Physical exam. A physical exam is crucial, but it may not be available for all adolescents. The goal of the physical exam should be to try to determine the etiology of the pain and exclude all other causes. For an adolescent who is not sexually active, a rectal abdominal exam can be performed. A common finding on pelvic exam in these patients includes cul-de-sac tenderness.[8]

Imaging. Pelvic ultrasound remains a cornerstone in the diagnosis of endometriosis, although it is less helpful in adolescents as endometrioma is rare in adolescents. An MRI examination is a better diagnostic tool, but the elevated cost makes it less accessible. [8]

Management

The first-line therapy in adolescents with endometriosis or where endometriosis is suspected is made by OCPs and NSAIDs. Unfortunately, many of these patients do not respond to this therapy and alternative options include GnRH analogues (only in patients over

140 | ADOLESCENTS AND ENDOMETRIOSIS

18 years) or laparoscopy. The use of GnRH agonists during adolescence is controversial, due to reported impacts on bone mass, and the same concern applies to GnRH antagonists.[2,10,11] A 2007 study on 36 adolescents between 13 and 21 years old showed that the use of norethindrone acetate as addback therapy, in adolescents treated with a GnRH agonist for endometriosis improves skeletal health. Laparoscopy remains the fundamental diagnostic tool for endometriosis when pharmacological treatment is not successful. Operative laparoscopy allows for a definitive diagnosis and treatment of endometriosis.[12,13] The procedure should be performed by a gynecologist, who is comfortable working with females at such a young age, as well as expert on the disease and its multifocality.[12] A clear understanding of the difference of endometriotic lesions in adolescents compared to those of adult women is needed. In teenagers, red lesions are predominant with atypical or white color, but rarely blue or brown lesions found in older patients. In young patients, surgical treatment alone in these cases is not considered appropriate, because microscopic residual disease may persist. Therefore, medication is often recommended after surgical therapy to prevent recurrences. In fact, younger age has been shown as an independent risk factor to endometriosis recurrence after conservative surgical treatment of endometriosis.[14,15]

What can parents do to help their teenagers manage severe pain related to endometriosis?[11]

- Get good information about pelvic pain.
- Recognize the effects of pain on your adolescent's thoughts and emotions.

ENDOMETRIOSIS | 141

- Help your daughter develop a support team (this may include gynecologist, pediatrician, relatives, friends, teachers, and the school nurse).
- Encourage your adolescent to go to school and maintain their social network. Also lead as normal a life as possible.
- Shift the focus away from pain.
- Help your adolescent develop a plan to manage a bad pain day.

An early diagnosis of endometriosis in the adolescent and prompt treatment reduces the risk of future ramifications, such as multiple laparoscopies during adulthood, the need for assisted reproduction technologies, and a loss of quality of life. In fact, for young patients, endometriosis as a chronic disease often negatively impacts their social and scholastic conditions.

Furthermore, adolescents with severe pelvic pain have a high rate of endometriosis. Thus, endometriosis should be strongly considered in adolescent females with pelvic pain. As such, timely referral to a gynecologist who is experienced with endometriosis, is an imperative, along with willingness to provide patient centered- care which may significantly benefit their future quality of life.[4,8,16]

Take Away

Severe Painful Periods During Adolescence Isn't Normal.

Power Point

An early diagnosis of endometriosis and prompt treatment reduce the risk of future sequelae.

CHAPTER XV
DISTANT ENDOMETRIOSIS

Distant or extra-pelvic endometriosis is a rare type of endometriosis that occurs in a distant site from gynecological organs and can be found in virtually every organ system and tissue in the body. This includes the lungs, heart, gallbladder, liver, small bowel, appendix, colon, rectum, kidney, and bladder. The umbilicus (navel), abdominal wall incisions, episiotomy scars, biceps muscle and bone, are other reported sites. Interestingly, the spleen has not been a site of reported endometriosis, which may be a factor in the origin and development of extra-pelvic endometriosis.[1] Endometriosis can occur in more than one place in the same patient and with extra-pelvic endometriosis, it usually does.

Depending on the location of endometrial tissue implantation, endometriosis can present with a wide variety of symptoms, making the diagnosis of distant endometriosis even more challenging. The consequence is likely an even greater delay in the diagnosis than pelvic endometriosis as it is neither easy nor routine. Many diagnostic methods, both clinical and laboratory, have been used in this process. However, none of them displays the gold standard. Extra-pelvic endometriosis should be cogently considered in patients who, present with a wide range of clinical issues such as cyclic hemoptysis (the coughing up blood), nausea or vomiting, hematuria (blood in the urine), and other symptoms during menses.[2] Regarding treatment, the approach is correlated with where the bulk of endometriosis is located. Accordingly, the treatment can vary from simple observation to surgical treatment, as well as treatment with medication and a combination of those.

Common Locations of endometriosis

Intestinal Endometriosis: is the most common location of extra-pelvic endometriosis with the urinary system being second.[3] Relevant to gastrointestinal endometriosis, the most prevalent bowel symptoms are rectal bleeding and pain. Others are painful bowel movements, loss of appetite, cramping, abdominal pains, and nausea and vomiting. Additionally, constipation and/ or diarrhea, abdominal bloating and gas are also associated with intestinal endometriosis. Moreover, these symptoms tend to get worse during menstruation. Aside from this the prevailing location of extra-pelvic intestinal endometriosis is the last part of the ileum (the small intestine), along with the cecum (the first part of the large bowel), and the appendix [2,4,5]

Case History: *Mildred, P,* is a 35-year-old female who presented to the emergency room with a history of lower abdominal pain and vomiting for over a month. She was being managed by her primary care physician for gastroenteritis and had a history of endometriosis diagnosed via laparoscopy. She had been prescribed a low-dose oral contraceptive but had discontinued the medication one month earlier. Her laboratory studies were normal, a barium enema showed a mass in the sigmoid colon. Colonoscopy demonstrated a tumor in the sigmoid colon with ulceration. Biopsy showed no evidence of malignancy or inflammatory bowel disease. She subsequently underwent laparoscopic sigmoidectomy, and the tissue pathology confirmed intestinal endometriosis with accompanying colitis. She was treated with a GnRH antagonist, and her quality of life improved significantly. No recurrence of the symptoms occurred during the six months of follow up. [4]

Urinary Tract Endometriosis: is the second most common site of extra-pelvic endometriosis. The predominate symptoms are local pain and cyclic hematuria (blood in the urine). Bladder and ureteral involvement are the most common sites, with the former representing 80–90% and the latter up to 50% of cases. Kidney and urethral endometriosis are extremely rare entities, with an incidence of 4% and 14%, respectively.[2] Women with urinary tract endometriosis are usually in their 30's or 40's. and half of them have had prior pelvic surgery. There are also several reports of bladder endometriosis arising after a cesarean section. Estrogen replacement therapy has been implicated in increasing the likelihood of developing urinary tract endometriosis. Regarding treatment, surgical excision of the endometriotic tissue, is the ideal treatment for all types of extra-pelvic endometriosis. Parenthetically, adjunctive treatment might be useful in selected cases.[3,6,7]

Case History: *Heidi, G* is a 25-year-old female who presented with a complaint of cyclical pelvic pain. The pain was stated to occur with her menses and usually lasted ten days. It commenced approximately six months prior to the evaluation and was described as

146 | Distant Endometriosis

severe and occurring in the lower abdomen area. She also complained about dysuria (burning with urination) and low back pain but denied a history of hematuria (blood in the urine). She had been evaluated by several gynecologists without relief. The abdominal examination was normal, save for the healed cesarian section scar. The pelvic examination was noted to be normal. Laboratory test results were negative, which included a urinalysis and urine culture. Pelvic ultrasound showed a mass related to the posterior bladder wall. The uterus and ovaries were normal in size. Office cystoscopy revealed a mass on the posterior wall of bladder. Transurethral resection was scheduled, and the mass was completely resected. The pathology specimen demonstrated endometriosis. She was placed on a GnRH agonist for six months post the procedure. In the first year of follow-up, she had not experienced any signs of recurrence of symptoms. Additionally pelvic ultrasound did not detect any lesions or masses.[6]

Thoracic Endometriosis: is a clinical entity that includes the presence of displaced endometrial tissue. It involves the pleura (a thin layer that covers the lungs and lines the chest cavity), the pericardium (the membrane enclosing the heart) and rarely the diaphragm (a muscular membranous partition separating the abdomen from the thorax and functions in respiration). This is often expressed as catamenial (menstrual) pneumothorax (air leaks into the space be-tween the lungs and chest wall). Catamenial pneumothorax is the most common clinical expression of thoracic endometriosis syndrome, which includes four other entities. These are in brief, catamenial hemothorax (a collection of blood in the space between the chest wall and the lung) catamenial hemoptysis (the coughing up blood), endometriotic lung nodules, and catamenial chest pain. The catamenial character of all these symptoms mentioned above is related to the menstrual cycle. More specifically, for the development of catamenial pneumothorax the presence of endometrial tissue in the thoracic cavity is necessary.[8,9,10]

Case History: *Sharon, J* is a thirty-seven-year-old with a history of three non-eventful spontaneous vaginal deliveries. Post her last delivery she received a tubal ligation. Additionally, she admits to experiencing extremely painful menstrual cramps and lower right sided abdominal pain, along with low back pain, right shoulder pain, nausea, and similar symptoms between periods. However, the symptoms between periods were not quite as intense. Unfortunately, her symptoms increased along with monthly right chest pain and shortness of breath (SOB). She frequented the emergency room for the complaints. However, the emergency room visits were all essentially the same. They acknowledge her symptoms; the labs and imaging were negative. She was discharged and advised to receive follow-up evaluation by her gynecologist. The follow-up evaluations by her gynecologist were without resolution. She changed gynecologist and then again. The third gynecologist placed her on oral contraceptives which gave her some relief for a few months. However, the symptoms were still disturbing. Her evaluation at another emergency room visit revealed a pneumothorax (air leaks into the space between the lungs and chest wall). She eventually received a thoracoscopic procedure (a procedure to look at the space inside of the chest, outside of the lungs). The procedure did not reveal the cause of the problem and biopsies was stated to be benign. She was referred to her gynecologist for treatment and follow-up. Who informed her that she had catamenia (menstrual) pneumothorax and advised her to have a hysterectomy. She received the hysterectomy with removal of her fallopian tubes and ovaries after which she was placed on hormonal replacement therapy.

Months post the hysterectomy she noted decreased abdominal and back pain. However, the chest pain, and SOB occurred off and on. Due to this she was referred to another gynecologist by a friend. The gynecologist reviewed her case in its entirety. He concluded that she had endometriosis which caused the pelvic pain, SOB, chest pain and pneumothorax. Her hormonal replacement medication was discontinued, and she was placed on medication (aromatase inhibitor). Twelve months later at one of her offices visits she stated, *"I feel wonderful."* Thus, she was finally able to find out, *"the name of her pain, endometriosis,"* and get relief.[11,12,13]

Treatment

The therapeutic options in the treatment of endometriosis depend on the extent of the disease, the patient's needs and the desire to maintain reproductive capacity. These options include:

- Simple observation,
- Surgical treatment,
- Medical treatment and
- Combined therapy.

In the past the simple observation without any intervention was considered appropriate for the initial stages of the disease, particularly, when minimal symptoms were present. Today therapeutic intervention after diagnosis of endometriosis is necessary, because the lesion of the disease usually increase with time. Conservative surgical treatment applies to patients who wish to preserve their reproductive capacity. This may include removal or destruction (laser ablation, electrocautery, thermal coagulation) of surface lesions or endometriomas (cysts); as well as lysing of adhesions and restoring normal anatomy. The surgical treatment of the disease is either via laparoscopy or laparotomy (open surgery). Regardless of the surgical technique (laparoscopy or laparotomy), removal of all endometrial lesions with careful lysing of adhesions is preferred. This has been found to be advantageous, especially relevant in redressing pelvic pain and infertility in women who wish to preserve their reproductive ability.[8,12,14]

Medical Treatment

Theoretically, medical treatment would be ideal in the treatment of endometriosis. In practice, however, drug therapy alone is accompanied with a temporary improvement of pain. The symptoms are abated but in time they usually return. Also, drug therapy can certainly reduce the size of endometriomas and facilitate their removal via surgery. Oral contraceptives are one of the main drug treatments and can cause a reduction of the quantity of blood during menses. Furthermore, they also reduce pain during the menstrual period. Additionally, there's a plenitude of safe and effective medications for endometriosis. Some of them are gonadotropin releasing hormone (GnRH) agonists and the newer gonadotropin releasing hormone (GnRH) antagonists. They block the production of ovarian-stimulating hormones, lowering estrogen levels and preventing menstruation. This causes endometrial tissue to regress. GnRH agonists and antagonists can force endometriosis into remission during the time of treatment and sometimes for months or years afterwards. The

150 | DISTANT ENDOMETRIOSIS

effectiveness of drug therapy on reproductive capacity is questionable. That is why drug therapy is often not recommended as the sole treatment of women with endometriosis, except for rare cases where surgery is not possible. This is also applicable to cases where surgery will present a significant risk to the life of the patient.[1,12]

Combination Therapy

The most effective way to treat endometriosis is via the combination of surgical removal of all visible endometrial lesions, in concert with the utilization of medication post the procedure.[8]

The endometrium is one of the most extraordinary tissues of the human body. It can be implanted in different tissues while maintaining its functionality, which explains the variety of symptoms that are components of the "endometriosis syndrome." Pain is the main symptom of endometriosis, but not the only one. Only the catamenial character of the symptoms can be considered as more indicative of endometriosis. Lastly, endometriosis is a common clinical entity even in its extra-pelvic form. Every clinician should have a high suspicion of it, particularly in cases of women with periodical symptoms. The importance of high clinical suspicion is critical relevant to the diagnosis and effectiveness of the treatment.

CHAPTER XVI
CLINICAL TRIALS

S cience is only as good as the evidence upon which it is based. Since medical science has such a vital effect on our health, it is important that every decision is based on strong clinical evidence. This evidence is provided by clinical trials and research. The National Institutes of Health (NIH) describe clinical trials as "research studies that explore whether a medical strategy, treatment, or device is safe and effective for humans." In this regard clinical trials often look for both healthy participants and individuals with specific conditions.[1]

Importance of Clinical Trials. Clinical trials provide us with details about the effectiveness and safety of a clinical intervention. Many clinical trials help researchers come up with better treatment strategies for a certain disease. Thus, some clinical trials compare two treatment methods to find out which one is better and safer. Clinical trials don't study just the newest medications or interventions; they may be used to study the long-term effects of drugs and interventions that are already in common use. For example, recent clinical trials have found that some hormonal therapies, which are already

152 | CLINICAL TRIALS

widely used may increase the risk of heart disease, stroke, blood clots and breast cancer. As a result, long-term use of hormonal therapy is recommended with caution in postmenopausal women.

Reasons for Conducting Clinical Trials. In general, clinical studies are designed to add to medical knowledge related to the treatment, diagnosis, and prevention of diseases or conditions. Some common reasons for conducting clinical studies include:

- Evaluating one or more interventions (for example, drugs, medical devices, approaches to surgery or radiation therapy) for treating a disease, syndrome, or condition.
- Finding ways to prevent the initial development or recurrence of a disease or condition. These can include medicines, vaccines, or lifestyle changes, among other approaches.
- Evaluating one or more interventions aimed at identifying or diagnosing a particular disease or condition.
- Examining methods for identifying a condition or the risk factors for that condition.
- Exploring and measuring ways to improve the comfort and quality of life through supportive care for people with a chronic illness.[1]

Clinical Trials. In a clinical trial, participants receive specific interventions according to the research plan or protocol. These interventions may be medical products, such as drugs or devices. They can also be procedures; or changes to participants' behavior, such as diet. Clinical trials may compare a new medical approach to a standard one that is already available; to a placebo that contains no active ingredients, or to no intervention. Some clinical trials compare interventions that are already available to each other. When a new product or approach is being studied. it is not usually known whether it will be helpful, harmful, or no different than available alternatives (including no intervention). The investigators try to determine the safety and efficacy of the intervention by measuring certain outcomes in the participants. For example, investigators may give a drug or treatment to participants who have high blood pressure to see whether their blood pressure decreases.[3,4]

Phases of Clinical Trials

Clinical trials are divided into phases. Each phase has different objectives and questions to answer. Scientists usually start a clinical trial on humans only after they have found a particular medication or intervention is effective in a laboratory or through animal studies. According to the FDA, clinical trials are carried out in four phases, with each phase building upon the knowledge gained from the prior phase. If the trial fails to fulfill its objective, it may be terminated.

Phase I Clinical Trial

Generally carried out in a very small group of people (usually 20-100 healthy subjects). The main objective of this trial is to understand safety, and safe dosages in humans.

Phase II Clinical Trial

In this phase, the trial is carried out on a larger group of people (several hundred people), and the objective is to know more about the effectiveness of medication or intervention, along with a collection of additional safety data.

Phase III Clinical Trial

Once the drug or intervention has been found safe and effective, it is tested on a much larger group of humans (usually few thousand) over the period of few years. If found effective and safe enough, it is given a marketing approval by FDA.

Phase IV Clinical Trial

The final phase, involving several thousand individuals suffering from the condition for which intervention or medication is being tested. Tests focus on the efficacy and safety on a much larger scale and in real life conditions.

It is also important to understand that not all clinical trials involve the study of new medications or interventions. For example, the genetic study of a group that suffers from a certain disease, or effect of living conditions on cardiac health.[5]

Response to Clinical Trial Concerns and Questions

Who Conducts Clinical Trials? Every clinical study is led by a principal investigator, who is usually a medical doctor. Clinical studies also have a research team that may include physicians, nurses, and other health care professionals.

Clinical trials can be sponsored, or funded, by pharmaceutical companies, academic medical centers, voluntary groups, and other organizations. In addition to Federal agencies such as the National Institutes of Health, the U.S. Department of Defense, and the U.S.

Department of Veterans Affairs. Physicians, other health professionals, and other individuals can also sponsor clinical research.

Where Are Clinical Trials Conducted? Clinical trials can take place in many locations, including hospitals, universities, physicians' offices, and community clinics. The location depends on who is conducting the study.

How Long Do Clinical Trials Last? The length of a clinical study varies, depending on what is being studied. Participants are told how long the study will last before they enroll.

Clinical Trial Participation. A clinical study is conducted according to a research plan known as the protocol. The protocol is designed to answer specific research questions and safeguard the health of participants. It contains the following information:

- The reason for conducting the study
- Who may participate in the study (the eligibility criteria)
- The number of participants needed
- The schedule of tests, procedures, or drugs and their dosages
- The length of the study
- What information will be gathered about the participants[1,2]

Who Can Participate in a Clinical Trial? Clinical studies have standards outlining who can participate. These standards are called eligibility criteria and are listed in the protocol. Some research studies seek participants who have the illnesses or conditions that will be studied, while other studies are looking for healthy participants. Ad-ditionally, some studies are limited to a predetermined group of people who are asked by researchers to enroll.

156 | CLINICAL TRIALS

Eligibility. The factors that allow someone to participate in a clinical study are called inclusion criteria, and the factors that disqualify someone from participating are called exclusion criteria. They are based on characteristics such as age, gender, the type and stage of a disease, previous treatment history, and other medical conditions.

How Are Participants Protected? Informed, consent is a process used by researchers to provide potential and enrolled participants with information about a clinical study. This information helps people decide whether they want to enroll or continue to participate in the study. The informed consent process is intended to protect participants and should provide enough information for a person to understand the risks or potential benefits, along with the alternatives to the research study. In addition to the informed consent document, the process may involve recruitment materials and may include verbal instructions, question-and-answer sessions, and activities to measure participant understanding. In general, a person must sign an informed consent document before joining a study. This is necessary to show that they were given information on the risks, potential benefits, and alternatives and to help display that they understand it. Signing the document and providing consent is not a contract. Participants may withdraw from a study at any time, even if the study is not over.

Institutional Review Boards. Each federally supported or conducted clinical study and each study of a drug, biological product, or medical device regulated by FDA. must be reviewed. It must also be approved and monitored by an institutional review board (IRB). An IRB is made up of physicians, researchers, and members of the community. Its role is to make sure that the study is ethical and that the rights and welfare of participants are protected. This includes making sure that research risks are minimized and are reasonable, particularly in relation to any potential benefits, among other responsibilities. The IRB also reviews the informed consent document.

In addition to being monitored by an IRB, some clinical studies are also monitored by data monitoring committees (also called data safety and monitoring boards).

Various Federal agencies, including the Office of Human Subjects Research Protection and FDA, have the authority to determine whether sponsors of certain clinical studies are adequately protecting research participants.[3,4]

Relationship to Usual Health Care. Typically, participants continue to see their usual physician or other health care professional while enrolled in a clinical study. While most clinical studies provide participants with medical products or interventions related to the illness or condition being studied, they do not provide extended or complete health care. By having his or her usual health care professional work with the research team, a participant can make sure that the study protocol will not conflict with other medications or treat-ments that he or she receive.

Considerations for Participation. Participating in a clinical study contributes to medical knowledge. The results of these studies can make a difference in the care of future patients by providing information about the benefits and risks of therapeutic, preventative, or diagnostic products or interventions.

158 | CLINICAL TRIALS

Clinical trials provide the basis for the development and marketing of new drugs, biological products, and medical devices. Sometimes, the safety and the effectiveness of the experimental approach or use may not be fully known at the time of the trial. Some trials may provide participants with the prospect of receiving direct medical benefits, while others do not. Most trials involve some risk of harm or injury to the participant, although it may not be greater than the risks related to routine medical care or disease progression. (For trials approved by IRBs, the IRB has decided that the risks of participation have been minimized and are reasonable in relation to anticipated benefits.) Many trials require participants to undergo additional procedures, tests, and assessments based on the study protocol. These requisites will be described in the informed consent document. A potential participant should also discuss these issues with members of the research team and with his or her usual healthcare professional.[5,6]

Questions to Ask. Anyone interested in participating in a clinical study should know as much as possible about the study, it is imperative that they feel comfortable asking the research team questions about the study, the related procedures, and any expenses. The following questions may be helpful during such a discussion. Answers to some of these questions are provided in the informed consent document.

- Ask about the purpose of the clinical trial.
- What will I have to do?
- What tests and procedures are involved?
- How often will I have to visit the study site?
- How long will the study last?

- Who will pay for my participation?
- Will I be reimbursed for other expenses?
- If I benefit from the intervention, will I be allowed to continue receiving it after the trial ends?
- Will results of the study be provided to me?
- Who will oversee my medical care while I am participating in the trial?

Why Participate in Clinical Trials? Everyone has different reasons to participate in a clinical trial. Healthy subjects mostly participate because they think that it is their duty to help science in moving forward. Many people suffering from diseases may participate in the hopes of getting better or cured. There are many medical conditions for which there is currently no effective treatment, such as different kinds of cancers.

There are certain eligibility criteria to decide who can participate in every clinical trial. Some trials require the participation of older people, while others focus on younger adults. Some may need healthy volunteers while others need patients with a particular disease condition. Trials may also vary in duration and location where they would be carried out. In some trials, a person may need to travel or stay at the medical facility.[2]

Response to Other Clinical Trial Concerns and Questions

The Benefits of Participating in a Clinical Trial. Benefits depend upon the phase or type of clinical trial. Clinical trials provide a person early access to the latest developments in the field of medicine. An individual may also get attention from the best specialists in their field, along with potentially better diagnostics. Apart from the possibility of direct health benefits, individuals get an opportunity to play a role in the development of science.

How Safe are Clinical Trials? There, is no guarantee that a person would benefit from a clinical trial, and some interventions or medications may cause unforeseen and severe side effects. Individuals are informed about the possible risks when signing the informed consent. It is also important to know that informed consent is not a contract, and a person can withdraw from the study at any given time.

Endometriosis Medical Research. There is a great deal of endometriosis research still to be done. Recent endometriosis clinical trials have focused on investigational treatments that may inhibit tissue growth and deactivate the chemical signaling mechanisms that promote overgrowth.

Why Are More Endometriosis Clinical Trials Necessary? Endometriosis clinical trials are essential to understanding the underlying causes of the disease. New clinical resources for endometriosis will require ardent investigation of the environmental and genetic factors that may predispose a patient to this condition. Endometriosis is classified into four stages depending on its severity and later stages can cause complications due to lesions, scarring, adhesions, tissue destruction, adverse anatomical changes, and cystic formation in the ovaries. Explicitly endometriosis clinical trials are sorely needed to define treatment protocols for each of these stages.[7]

In summary, reduced diagnosis of endometriosis has led to it remaining a relatively mysterious condition. Millions of women suffer from endometriosis including those who do not know it yet. With investigational endometriosis treatments, new endometriosis clinical resources may finally be on the way. Parenthetically, any woman who has suffered from the disease or has a relative who does, has a role to play.[7,8]

Take Away

Women who have endometriosis should consider participating in clinical trials.

CHAPTER XVII
CASE HISTORIES OF ENDOMETRIOSIS

Endometriosis presents itself differently in various women and can also co-occur with other conditions. Therefore, every case of endometriosis should be treated as unique and personalized. Despite the differences, there are certain commonalities among cases, which is why this section aims to provide examples of the more common endometriosis scenarios. The goal is to help individuals better understand their own situation.

Case History 1: Endometriosis and Fibroids

WJ is a 40-year-old with a long history of right sided pelvic pain, which occurs during her menses along with heavy periods, both of which increased a few months prior to her evaluation. She was evaluated by her gynecologist, who noted that her complaints included nausea, diarrhea, and lower back pain with her periods. The pelvic examination revealed an enlarged uterus (12 weeks pregnancy size which is equivalent to the size of a grapefruit). An ultrasound was ordered which noted several uterine fibroid tumors. The laboratory

164 | CASE HISTORIES OF ENDOMETRIOSIS

studies demonstrated anemia. She received an office hysteroscopy which did not reveal fibroids in the uterine cavity. The tissue from the endometrial biopsy done at the same time was benign. The gynecologist's impression was uterine fibroids which was the cause of the heavy periods and anemia, as well as endometriosis (clinical diagnosis), which was responsible for the right sided pelvic pain during the periods, as well as low back pain, nausea, and diarrhea. After her consultation with a review of the findings, she received medical and surgical options. The surgical options were laparoscopy, with possible C02 laser treatment of endometriosis with myomectomy or hysterectomy. The medical options were with one of the new GnRH antagonists' combination medications. The patient did not want surgery and choose the GnRH antagonist combination. After three months on the medication, she experienced minimal bleeding and pain with her periods. The fibroids were also slightly smaller via an ultrasound evaluation.

Case History 2: Endometriosis and Polycystic Ovaries

JA is a 26-year-old who complained about severe cramps with infrequent periods. However, when she did have her period, they are extremely heavy with large blood clots that often lasts for weeks. She was given birth control pills to control the problem, but when she discontinued them to get pregnant, the problem not only persisted but became worse.

An evaluation by her new gynecologist noted facial hair, and that she was overweight. The pelvic exam revealed a normal size uterus with scarring and tenderness. Her laboratory tests were within normal limits. The pelvic ultrasound noted large polycystic ovaries. The gynecologist's diagnosis was polycystic ovaries syndrome which was responsible for the infrequent periods as well as a clinical diagnosis of endometriosis, which was responsible for her pelvic pain during her menses. The exam also noted pelvic tenderness and scarring. Both the endometriosis and polycystic ovaries can be responsible for her not getting pregnant.

The gynecologist recommended robotic surgery, (laparoscopy) with CO_2 laser to ascertain the extent of endometriosis, stage it and treat, it. Along with this, CO_2 laser ovarian drilling was advised to treat the polycystic ovaries. Hysteroscopy was also recommended. The patient received the procedures wherein stage III endometriosis was noted. The endometriosis was treated along with the polycystic ovaries with CO_2 laser. Her husband's semen analysis was within normal limits. She received ovulation induction with an aromatase inhibitor and became pregnant three months after the procedure.

Case History 3: Endometriosis and Post Hysterectomy Pain

ES is a 43-year-old who underwent an abdominal hysterectomy three year ago for pelvic pain. However, a year after the hysterectomy the pain persisted. As a result, she underwent a laparoscopic bilateral salpingooophorectomy (removal of the fallopian tubes and ovaries). Nevertheless, the pain persisted, wherein she consulted several gynecologists without clear answers. Finally, she was evaluated by another gynecologist who opined that the pain was due to endometriosis. The evaluation revealed that she was taking hormonal replacement medication i.e., estrogen for hot flashes.

166 | CASE HISTORIES OF ENDOMETRIOSIS

Additionally, she had lower abdominal and pelvic tenderness. The pelvic ultrasound was unremarkable, and the laboratory studies were within normal limits. She was given options to diagnosis and possibly treat the pain: medication versus laparoscopy. She opted for laparoscopy and underwent the procedure. The surgeon noted endometriosis biopsied, excised and treated it with C02 laser. The patient did exceptionally well post-procedure with minimal occasional discomfort.

Case History 4: Endometriosis and Adenomyosis

ME, is a 38 year with severe mid and left lower abdominal pain with her periods. She also experienced heavy menstrual bleeding, which increased after having her fourth child four years ago. Initially, she was given birth control pills, which provided relief, but she no longer desired to take them. She was offered a hysterectomy as a solution but did not want to undergo that type of procedure. A second opinion evaluation noted a large boggy and tender uterus. The pelvic ultrasound revealed findings consistent with adenomyosis. An MRI also showed presumptive adenomyosis and endometriosis. She decided to have laparoscopy to determine the extent of endometriosis and hysteroscopy to evaluate the heavy menstrual bleeding. The laparoscopy revealed stage II endometriosis with adhesions and scarring. The endometriosis was excised, adhesions lysed, and the patient received one of the new GnRH antagonists for endometriosis, which eliminated the bleeding problem.

Case History 5: Endometriosis and Infertility

HW, is a 28-year teacher who has been married for three years and had been trying to conceive for the past two years. Her husband is 32, healthy and has a normal semen analysis. She has a long history of severe menstrual cramps, painful intercourse, low back pain, and nausea with her periods, for which she has routinely taken ibuprofen and other medications. She has also taken different types of birth control pills for years and discontinued them to get pregnant. She decided to consult her friend's gynecologist, who noted a negative history for medical illnesses or surgery. The physical exam was normal including the pelvic exam. An ultrasound was also normal. However, a hysterosalpingogram revealed that her fallopian tubes were not blocked. In addition, the laboratory studies were normal. A review of the factors for infertility, which include male, cervix, endometrial, ovarian, tubal, peritoneal, and endocrine factors were negative. She received a clinical diagnosis of endometriosis which was stated to be responsible for the pelvic pain and infertility. Her gynecologist recommended laparoscopy to diagnosis and treat the problems. The laparoscopy revealed stage II, endometriosis with endometriotic lesions particularly on the right side. The lesions were excised, and she became pregnant two months after the procedure.

Case History 6: Endometriosis and Post-Menopausal Pain

MM is a 55-year-old who realized menopause two years ago. Prior to that she experienced generalized lower abdominal and back pain for years which was primarily associated with her periods. However, she also experienced pain between periods and around the time of ovulation. Due to the disturbing hot flashes, she received hormonal replacement therapy shortly after menopause. She documented that this was the time when the lower abdominal pain became worse. The hormonal replacement medication was discontinued however, the pain persisted. The physical exam was within normal limits as was the pelvic exam. Except for tenderness and scarring on both sides of the uterus. A pelvic ultrasound was negative as was the laboratory studies. Following a review of the options she decided to have laparoscopy, which revealed stage II endometriosis. The endometriotic lesions were excised and treated with C02 laser. She felt better after the procedure and experienced less pain. She was also elated that she was able to find out *the name of her pain.*

Case History 7: Endometriosis and Ovarian Cyst

AW is a 25-year-old who is on birth control pills mainly for severe cramps. However, they are working less than in the past. In fact, even after switching pills, recently she experienced pain when she was not on her period. Disturbingly, the pain became so intense on her left side that she went to the emergency room. The evaluation revealed an ovarian cyst which was confirmed via pelvic ultrasound. She was then referred to a gynecologist. who highlighted her history of severe cramps, nausea, and frequent stools with her periods. Added to this a family history of endometriosis. The physical exam was within normal limits. The pelvic examination however revealed left side tenderness and a mass. A repeat ultrasound noted an ovarian cyst (presumptive endometrioma or chocolate cyst). Her laboratory studies demonstrated slight elevation of CA 125 (a blood test that may be elevated in certain patients with endometriosis). She received laparoscopy for the pain and cyst, which confirmed endometriosis and chocolate cyst of the left ovary. The cyst was removed, and endometriosis was otherwise excised and ablated. She was also placed on one of the new GnRH antagonists for six months. Months later she was completely satisfied, stating, *"I feel like a new person."*

Therefore, as stated, these *"case histories"* should hopefully provide a better understanding of endometriosis and its various presentations, which can include co-occurrence with other disorders and a range of adverse effects. It is crucial to continue researching, studying, sharing information, and seeking out an endometriosis specialist or gynecologist, who is knowledgeable and compassionate in providing appropriate treatment options for patients with endometriosis.

CHAPTER XVIII
ENDOMETRIOSIS AWARENESS

It's impossible to talk about *"endometriosis awareness,"* without mentioning Mary Lou Ballweg. She is a paragon and a host of other complimentary adjectives. Ballweg is president and executive director of the Endometriosis Association, an organization she helped found in 1980. Besides founding and leading the association for the last forty plus years. She has overseen publication of the association's two books, educational videotapes, together with as an extensive body of literature on endometriosis. She has also overseen the development and execution of a $1.3 million educational awareness campaign, along with two public service announcement campaigns, as well as numerous other outreach efforts. Ballweg helped found the world's first research registry for endometriosis. She was also responsible for a breakthrough in endometriosis research, which linked the condition to dioxin. This breakthrough received attention in leading scientific journals, prompting numerous additional research studies. Further, Ballweg was instrumental in

172 | ENDOMETRIOSIS AWARENESS

establishing research programs for endometriosis at Dartmouth Medical School and Vanderbilt University School of Medicine.[1]

Endometriosis Awareness Month (EAM) is recognized in recognition of the estimated over 190 million women suffering from endometriosis.[2] Each March, millions worldwide observe Endometriosis Month. It began because the founding mother of, EAM, herself Mary Lou Ballweg, along with seven other women founded an Endometriosis Awareness Week. The Endometriosis Awareness Week was established during the Endometriosis Association's roundtable in Milwaukee. The group of eight soon grew to twenty-two and shortly after, the designated week took on a new life of its own. They could not do everything all around the world in just a week, so it was expanded to a month.[3]

March was chosen because it falls between two major climate issues (the very cold winter and the hot and humid summer). There was also the issue of separating the awareness time from other significant events. Ballweg noted that"Fall was a more difficult time because that is major, fundraising time, "Strength in Numbers." Endometriosis was stated to be a far more taboo topic just a few decades ago. As a result, Ballweg and her colleagues had to fight hard against ambivalence and ignorance.[4,5,6]

The Yellow Ribbon. Yellow is universally known to be the color for Endometriosis Awareness, but why? Yellow was established as the color for endometriosis starting in 1980 with the publishing of the first popular yellow brochure. Because it was yellow, written in so many languages, and distributed worldwide, yellow became the color of endometriosis. It is also related to the iniquitousness of the symbolic ribbon. Initially, the ribbon was initially plain and did not represent anything related to endometriosis. Thus, it was decided to put wording on it to raise awareness. The wording, *"Ask me about endometriosis"* was added and it became an awareness tool.[5,6]

Lastly, Ballweg has traveled the world, highlighting endometriosis by providing information and education through presentations and the proverbial yellow brochures. I am fortunate enough to have observed her energy and many talents at numerous medical conferences throughout the world. Additionally, I had the honor of traveling as a delegate circa 2001 via an Endometriosis Association Initiative as one of the two gynecologists, Ballweg and four endometriosis advocates. Our delegation traveled to various medical hospitals and institutions to engage health professionals throughout China. Our mission involved communicating, collaborating, and teaching, about endometriosis, particularly relevant to the contemporary diagnosis and treatment.

CHAPTER XIX
THE FUTURE

Viewing or predicting the future under any circumstances, can be perplexing and arduous. This task is even more onerous when dealing with a complex disease like endometriosis. As previously stated, endometriosis is an inflammatory chronic pain condition that is related to uterine tissue growing outside of the uterus, affecting at least 10% of women worldwide.

Endometriosis results in a substantial burden to the affected women and society at large despite being identified more than 160 years ago. Unfortunately, substantial knowledge gaps remain, including confirmation of the disease's etiology. Research funding for endometriosis is important; however, it is limited. For example, funding from bodies like the National Institute of Health (NIH) constituted only 0.38% of the 2022 health budget. This is concerning, given the condition affects 6.5 million women in the US and over 190 million worldwide[1] A major issue is that the diagnosis of endometriosis is frequently delayed partly due to the fact that surgery is required to confirm the diagnosis. Diagnosis is also dependent on the intraoperative presentation and the surgeon's skill and experience. It's

176 | THE FUTURE

clear that this delay increases symptom intensity and sensitization, which is compounded by the costs of the disease for the patient and their nation.

The current conservative treatments of presumed endometriosis are pain management and the use of oral contraceptives. However, both methods are patently flawed and can be entirely ineffective, particularly regarding the reduction of patient suffering or improvement in the ability to work. It is also true, that neither addresses the infertility issues or the higher risk of certain cancers. Obviously, endometriosis research deserves the funding and attention that befits a disease; that has such substantial prevalence, effects, and economic costs. This funding could improve patient outcomes by introducing less invasive and more timely methods, especially regarding diagnosis and treatment concerns. This could include options such as novel biomarkers, nanomedicine, and microbiome alternatives.[1,2]

Research Priorities

It is important to identify issues and problems relevant to endometriosis, particularly in creating a roadmap or plan to redress them. This is exactly what the UK and Ireland did in 2017 with the formation of the Endometriosis Priority Setting Partnership (PSP). The objective of the PSP was to identify the key questions about endometriosis, especially, those that were most important to both women with endometriosis and healthcare practitioners involved in their care.[3] The PSP included women with endometriosis, their supporters, key health-care practitioners, and endometriosis researchers, as well as representatives from organizations involved with women with endometriosis.

Research questions were gathered from women with endometriosis, health-care practitioners, and researchers using surveys, online voting, and a facilitated workshop that included equal numbers of women with endometriosis and health-care practitioners. They devised the UK and Ireland 2017 top ten research priorities for endometriosis. The ten priorities were intended to provide a platform for researchers, funding bodies and the pharmaceutical industry to ensure that future research funding and research activities focus on questions, that are important to women with endometriosis and to health-care practitioners. These priorities are still relevant today and can be altered or modified for other countries, including the US.[3]

The Top Ten Research Priorities for Endometriosis in the UK and Ireland [3]

1. Can a cure be developed for endometriosis?
2. What causes endometriosis?
3. What are the most effective ways of educating health-care professionals throughout the health-care system. Which may result in reduced time to diagnosis and improve treatment and care of women with endometriosis?
4. Is it possible to develop a non-invasive screening tool to aid the diagnosis of endometriosis?
5. What are the most effective ways of maximizing and/or maintaining fertility in women with confirmed or suspected endometriosis?
6. How can the diagnosis of endometriosis be improved?
7. What is the most effective way of managing the emotional and/or psychological and/or fatigue impact of living with

endometriosis (including medical, non-medical, and self-management methods)?

8. What are the outcomes and/or success rates for surgical or medical treatments that aim to cure or treat endometriosis, rather than manage it?

9. What is the most effective way of stopping endometriosis progressing and/or spreading to other organs (after surgery)?

10. What are the most effective non-surgical ways of managing endometriosis-related pain and/or symptoms (medical/non-medical)[3]

Evolving Possibilities

The utility of the top ten priorities is that they provide a phenomenal guide, which possibly offers answers for the resolution of some of the issues. Fortunately, there is a lot of promising research underway that could create substantial positive ramifications for patients. These include the chance for non-invasive biomarker auxiliary diagnostic methods, the application of nanoparticle drug delivery, and treatments targeting the microbiome, which provides immense potential for developing new non-invasive diagnostic and treatment options. Along with the opportunity for nanoparticles to deliver therapies directly to endometriotic lesions. In Addition, innovation in artificial intelligence (AI), machine learning (ML) and deep learning (DL) is emerging as a promising data-driven approach beneficial in solving various problems applicable to endometriosis. Thus, advancement in the identification and treatment of endometriosis is challenging but entirely possible.[1,4,5]

New Biomarker Analysis. One of the key aspects impacting the diagnosis and treatment of endometriosis is the lack of non-invasive diagnostic tools. Biomarkers present an appealing option for non-invasive diagnosis of endometriosis. More research is needed to locate biomarkers that can adequately diagnosis endometriosis.[1,6,7]

Nanomedicines. One technology in its infancy for the treatment of endometriosis is the use of nanoparticles. They aid in the imaging that allows the direct treatment or delivering drugs to treat endometriosis. Nanoparticles have shown a capacity to accumulate in endometriotic lesions, which could improve the use of imaging technologies to diagnose endometriosis. This technology could also provide methods for targeting endometriotic lesions, without the requirement of surgery. Various drugs may possibly reduce the size or eliminate endometriosis lesions, rather than just suppressing symptoms. However, much more pre-clinical and clinical research is required to support the use of this emerging technology for endometriosis.[1]

Alterations to the Microbiome. Imbalances to gut microbiota compositions have been shown to impact endometriosis. In addition to being a potential site for new biomarkers, the gut microbiota may be a target site for new treatments. Therapies that address endometriotic alteration to the gut microbiota could have an enormous potential to reduce the growth of lesions, along with the effects of inflammation for endometriosis patients.[1]

Artificial Intelligence, Machine Learning Deep Learning and Augmented Reality. In the past few years artificial intelligence (AI) has spread rapidly into healthcare. It has demonstrated marked

180 | THE FUTURE

potential in disease diagnostics, treatments, and higher-level analysis of large biomedical datasets. Given the diversity of its use in the clinical context, there is great potential to apply AI to the complex challenges presented by endometriosis. Furthermore, AI can improve non-invasive diagnostics to reduce the delays and human error associated with diagnosis.[8,9]

Currently the use of AI in imaging, particularly machine learning (ML), has become a reality in clinical practice. The use of AI in gynecologic ultrasound has been proposed for the evaluation of the uterus and automatic classification of ovarian cysts.

In the field of gynecological surgery, the use of augmented reality (AR) helps surgeons detect vital structures, thus, decreasing complications, reducing operative time, and helping surgeons in training to practice in a realistic setting. Using three-dimensional (3D) printers can provide materials that mimic real tissues and helps trainees to practice on a realistic model. Furthermore, 3D imaging allows better depth perception than its two-dimensional (2D) counterpart, which allows the surgeon to create preoperative plans according to tissue depth and dimensions.[6,10] Although AI has some limitations, this new technology can improve the prognosis and management of patients, reduce healthcare costs and help Ob/Gyn practitioners to reduce their workload; increase their efficiency and accuracy by incorporating AI systems into their daily practice. AI has the potential to guide practitioners in decision-making, reaching a diagnosis, and improving case management. It can reduce healthcare costs by decreasing medical errors and providing more dependable predictions. AI systems can accurately provide information on a large array of patients in clinical settings, although more robust data is required[11,12,13,1415,16,17,18]

There are many interesting possibilities in both research and treatment for the future. If endometriosis had more representative funding, the rate of advancement of non-invasive diagnostic and treatment methods could be significantly increased, providing long-term benefits for patients and society. So, let us hope as we move forward, we can provide the necessary resources to extend our understanding of endometriosis to abate its impact on women in the US and the rest of the world.[1,11]

Take Away

- The UK and Ireland Top Ten Endometriosis Priorities, provides a phenomenal guide to possibly redress some of the issues related to endometriosis.
- There is a lot of promising endometriosis research underway that could create substantial positive ramifications for women.
- If endometriosis had more representative funding, the rate of advancement of non-invasive diagnostic and treatment methods could be significantly increased?

CHAPTER XX
THE EPILOGUE

As we come to the end of "Endometriosis, The Name of the Pain and How to Repress It." I hope that you have gained valuable insight into this often misunderstood and underdiagnosed condition. Endometriosis is a chronic illness that affects millions of women worldwide, causing pain and infertility that can have a significant impact on their quality of life.

In this book, I have discussed the various symptoms of endometriosis, including the most common symptom, pain, as well as its relationship to infertility. I have also explored the potential role of environmental toxins in the development and progression of endometriosis. As well as it's connection with fibroid tumors and cancer.

The contemporary diagnosis and treatment options for endometriosis has been presented, including both traditional medical-surgical approaches and alternative treatments. It is important to note that while there is no cure for endometriosis, there are many ways to manage its symptoms and improve quality of life.

184 | THE EPILOGUE

I have also touched on the topic of clinical trials for endometriosis, which are crucial for advancing our understanding and improving treatment options for this condition. Additionally, I have discussed the unique challenges faced by adolescents with endometriosis and the potential risks of unnecessary hysterectomies in the treatment of this condition.

The exciting potential of artificial intelligence (AI) in the future of endometriosis diagnosis and treatment has been explored. Clearly, as technology continues to advance. We may be able to diagnose and treat endometriosis more accurately and effectively.

Finally, it's time to end the namelessness of endometriosis and reveal it to the world, in order to put an end to the havoc and destruction it causes. Also, it's imperative to talk about endometriosis with everyone you know, and pass this book on to family, friends and associates; encourage them to do the same. Additionally give it to your gynecologist or other healthcare professionals and start a discussion about the disease. Discuss endometriosis on social media and join an endometriosis support group such as the Endometriosis Association or start your own. It will take all of us, working together to make a difference.

I hope that this book has been informative and empowering, and that it will encourage more awareness and research into *"endometriosis, the name of the pain."* With continued efforts, we can" repress endometriosis," and improve the lives of those affected by this condition and move towards a brighter future for women's health.

APPENDIX

GLOSSARY

A

Ablation
Surgical removal or destruction of tissue via laser or other modalities.

Adenomyosis
Disease characterized by growth of the endometrium into the walls of the uterus.

Adhesions
Scar tissue that is formed by bleeding endometriosis lesions and surgery. This scar tissue can bind together internal organs and surfaces → Read more

Adjuvants
A therapy used in conjunction with another, i.e. hormonal treatment after surgery.

Adnexal mass
A mass in the area of the Fallopian tube or ovary.

Adnexal torsion
A twisting of ovary or, rarely, the Fallopian tube.

188 | GLOSSARY

Agonist

A chemical that binds to some receptor of a cell and triggers a response by that cell. Agonists often mimic the action of a naturally occurring substance.

Amenorrhea

Refers to a woman who is not having her period, either because of a medical condition or because her menstruation is being suppressed by drug treatment.

Analgesic

A drug to relieve pain.

Androgen

Male sex hormones.

Andrologist

A physician-scientist who performs laboratory evaluations of male fertility. May hold a PhD. Degree instead of an MD. Usually affiliated with a fertility treatment center working on in vitro fertilization.

Androstenedione

One of the androgens (male hormones) that are naturally present in women. (Other androgens include testosterone and DHEAS.) These hormones play an important role in ovulation. High levels of androgens in women may indicate an abnormality in the ovulation process.

Aneuploidy

The loss or gain of one or more chromosomes.

Anovulation

The failure to ovulate.

Antagonist

A drug or other substance that exerts an opposite action to that of another or competes for the same receptor sites. An estrogen antagonist, for example, blocks estrogen.

Antepartum

The pre-delivery pregnancy period.

Anterior

Top or upper.

Antibodies

Chemicals made by the body to fight or attack foreign substances entering the body. Normally they prevent infection; however, when they attack the sperm or fetus, they cause infertility. Sperm antibodies may be made by either the man or the woman.

Antigen

Any substance that when introduced into the body, is recognized by the immune system.

Antioxidants

Compounds in the body or in nutrients that slow or prevent the effects of harmful substances called free radicals by converting these free radicals into water and oxygen. Free radicals are highly reactive substances found in air pollution, tobacco smoke, pesticides, food and ultraviolet sunlight that are manufactured during normal body processes, they damage cell membranes and result in tissue damage associated with heart disease, cancer, arthritis, premature aging and other conditions,. Antioxidants help slow or prevent these processes and may play a role in the immune system. (*Nutrition for Women by Elizabeth Somer, New York, Henry Holt and Company, 1993*)

Apoptosis

"Cell suicide," a process by which a genetically damaged cell destroys itself.

Aromatase

Enzyme that converts adrenal hormones into estrogen in fat and in endometrial cells.

Artificial Insemination (AI)

The depositing of sperm in the vagina near the cervix or directly into the uterus, with the use of a syringe instead of by coitus. This technique is used to overcome sexual performance problems, to circumvent sperm-mucus interaction problems, to maximize the potential for poor semen, and for using donor sperm.

Artificial Intelligence

The collective attributes of computer, robot, or other mechanical device programmed to perform functions analogous to learning and decision making.

Asherman's Syndrome

A condition where the uterine walls adhere to one another. Usually caused by uterine inflammation.

Assisted hatching

Perforating the zona pellucida ('shell' of the egg) to help the very early embryo (the blastocyst) escape, i.e.. to hatch. Can be done by needle, by the use of an acid tyrodes, or by laser.

Assisted Reproductive Technology (ART)

The term used to describe several procedures employed to bring about conception without sexual intercourse, including IUI, IVF, GIFT and ZIFT.

Atrophy

Thinning and decreased blood flow to tissue resultant from a lack of hormones, most commonly estrogen.

Autoimmune Disorders

When a person has an autoimmune disorder, immune cells mistakenly attack the body's own cells. Examples of autoimmune disorders are lupus, rheumatoid arthritis, and Grave's Disease. Some autoimmune factors, such as antiphospholipid antibodies, may affect fertility or pregnancy.

B

Basal Body Temperature (BBT)

The body reaches a basal metabolic temperature early in the morning when we are at rest. Charting this temperature variation helps determine when ovulation occurs. The basal body temperature is measured with a special basal thermometer.

Benign

Noncancerous

Benign Tumor

Noncancerous, abnormal growth

Beta hCG Test

A blood test used to detect very early pregnancies and to evaluate embryonic development.

Bicornuate Uterus

A congenital malformation of the uterus where the upper portion (horn) is duplicated.

Bilateral salpingo-oophorectomy (BSO)

Removal of both ovaries and fallopian tubes.

192 | GLOSSARY

Biomarker

A physiological substance when present in abnormal amounts in the serum may indicate the presence of disease

Blastocyst

The very early embryo.

Bowel resection

A surgical procedure performed when a blockage of the intestines occurs. The procedure removes the portion of the bowel where the obstruction is located.

Brownfield

The term is also used to describe land previously used for industrial or commercial purposes with known or suspected pollution including soil contamination due to hazardous waste.

C

Catamenia

Menses.

Cauterize

To burn tissue with electrical current (electrocautery) or with a laser. Used in surgical procedures to remove unwanted tissue such as adhesions and endometriotic implants. Also used to control bleeding.

CBC (Complete Blood Count)

A routine blood test is that analyses the three major types of cells in blood: red blood cells, white blood cells, and platelets. A CBC is a general indicator of overall health.

Cervical Stenosis

A blockage of the cervical canal from a congenital defect or from complications of surgical procedures.

Cervix

The opening between the uterus and the vagina. The cervical mucus plugs the cervical canal and normally prevents foreign materials from entering the reproductive tract. The cervix remains closed during pregnancy and dilates during labor and delivery to allow the baby to be born.

Chemical pregnancy

Very early pregnancy that is indicated through a positive pregnancy test only. When the term is used in connection with IVF, a chemical pregnancy may not be a pregnancy at all, but rather the result of the hCG injection creating a false-positive pregnancy test.

Chlamydia

A sexually transmitted infection caused by the microorganism chlamydia trachomatis, which if left untreated in a woman may cause pelvic inflammatory disease (PID), pelvic adhesions, and tubal blockage.

Chocolate cyst (endometrioma)

A cyst in the ovary that is filled with old blood, also known as an endometrioma. It occurs when endometriosis invades an ovary.

Chromosome

The structures in the cell that carry the genetic material (genes); the genetic messengers of inheritance. The human has forty-six chromosomes, twenty-three coming from the egg and twenty-three coming from the sperm.

Cilia

Tiny hairlike projections lining the inside surface of the fallopian tubes. The waving action of these "hairs" sweeps the egg toward the uterus.

194 | GLOSSARY

Clinical pregnancy
Pregnancy in which the fetus shows on an ultrasound at about seven weeks.

Clitoris
The small erectile sex organ of the female which contains large numbers of sensory nerves, the female counterpart of the penis.

Clone
A perfect copy of a (DNA) molecule, a (stem) cell or an individual. Cloning of an individual is done by replacing the nucleus of an egg cell with the genetic material from a somatic (non-germ) cell – as was done to make Dolly the sheep, the world's first clone. Cloning can also be done to produce stem cells, the undifferentiated early cells from which all types of cells develop. This technique may in the future enable people to access life-saving treatments tailored-made from their own DNA.

Coagulation
A method of destroying endometrial lesions by dehydrating the cells with a bipolar or thermal coagulator.

Coelomic epithelium
Tissue in the embryo that develops into the lining of the pelvis.

Cohort
A 'cohort study' looks at groups of people, recording their exposure to certain risk factors to find clues as to the possible causes of disease. They can be forward-looking (prospective) or backward-looking (retrospective).

Coitus
Intercourse; the sexual union between a man and a woman.

Conception
The fertilization of an ovum or the act of becoming pregnant.

Contraceptives

Any agent or device used for the prevention of conception (getting pregnant).

Controlled ovarian hyperstimulation (COH)

Stimulation of multiple ovulations with fertility drugs; also known as superovulation.

Corpus luteum

The yellow-pigmented glandular structure that forms from the ovarian follicle following ovulation. The gland produces progesterone, which is responsible for preparing and supporting the uterine lining for implantation. Progesterone also causes the half-degree basal temperature elevation noted at mid-cycle during an ovulatory cycle. If the corpus luteum functions poorly, the uterine lining may not support a pregnancy. If the egg is fertilized, a corpus luteum of pregnancy forms to maintain the endometrial bed and support the implanted embryo. A deficiency in the amount of progesterone produced (or the length of time it is produced) by the corpus luteum can mean the endometrium is unable to sustain a pregnancy. This is called luteal phase defect (LPD).

Cul-de-sac

The space between the back of the uterus and the rectum that forms a pouch.

Cytokines

Powerful chemical substances secreted by immune cells.

Cryopreservation

Frozen storage of sperm, eggs, embryos, or other reproductive tissue for later use.

196 | GLOSSARY

Cyst
A closed bladder like sac containing fluid or semifluid matter such as an ovarian cyst.

D

D&C (Dilation and Curettage)
Surgical dilation of the cervix followed by surgical scraping of the interior of the uterine cavity with a curette (spoon-shaped surgical instrument) to remove growths (eg. pregnancy, tumors, etc) or diseased tissue.

Decidualization:
Is a process that results in significant changes to cells of the endometrium in preparation for and during pregnancy.

Deep Learning
An advanced type of machine learning architecture employed by neural networking most commonly by convolutional neural networks.

Delayed puberty
A condition in which the youngster fails to complete puberty and develop secondary sex characteristics by sixteen years of age. Puberty may be stimulated with hormonal replacement therapy. Some will outgrow the condition without treatment.

Denervation
Loss of neuronal connections.

DHEAS (dihydroeprandrostone)
One of the androgens (male hormones) that are naturally present in women. (Other androgens include testosterone and androstenedione.) These hormones play an important role in ovulation. High levels of androgens in women may indicate an abnormality in the ovulation process.

Dioxin

TCCDD (2,3,7,8-tetrachlorodibenzo-p-dioxin), the most toxic of a group of chemicals prevalent in the environment from herbicides, industrial wastes and other sources, dioxin is a toxic chemical by-product of pesticide manufacturing, bleached pulp and paper products and hazardous waste burning.

Diabetes

A condition in which the glucose (sugar) in the blood is too high because the body is unable to use it properly. Diabetes may be responsible for decreased fertility and increased incidence of miscarriage.

Disease

A disease is defined as any deviation from or interruption of the normal structure or function of any part, organ, or system, or combination thereof, of the body that is manifested by a characteristic set of symptoms or signs.

Dysmenorrhea

Painful menstruation. This may be a sign of endometriosis.

Dyspareunia

Painful intercourse.

E

Ectopic pregnancy

A pregnancy outside of the uterus, usually in the Fallopian tube.

Eggs

Female cells containing 23 chromosomes that are stored in the ovaries. When fertilized by sperm, an egg forms an embryo. A woman is born with all the eggs she will ever have. Each month, an egg is released during ovulation. If it is not fertilized, menstruation will occur about two weeks later.

During IVF fertility drugs are given, which cause the ovaries to produce numerous eggs instead of just one.

Egg retrieval

A procedure used to obtain eggs from ovarian follicles for use in in vitro fertilization (IVF). The procedure may be performed during laparoscopy or by using a long needle and ultrasound to locate the follicle in the ovary.

Embryo

The early products of conception, ie. the undifferentiated beginnings of a baby.

Embryo transfer

Placing an egg fertilized outside the womb into a woman's uterus or fallopian tube.

Empty Sella Syndrome

A condition that occurs when spinal fluid leaks into the bony chamber (fossa) housing the pituitary gland. The fluid pressure compresses the pituitary gland and may adversely affect its ability to secrete LH and FSH and may elevate prolactin levels.

Endometrial biopsy

A test to check for Luteal Phase Defect during which a sample of the uterine lining is collected for microscopic analysis. The biopsy results will confirm ovulation and the proper preparation of the endometrium by estrogen and progesterone stimulation.

Endometrial cells

The cells that make up the lining of the uterus. These cells build up a thick lining cyclically which is then discarded through menstrual flow.

Endometrial Implant

Small bluish, red, purple, white or clear areas/blebs that may be found in the pelvic region due to endometriosis.

Endometrioma (chocolate cyst)

A cyst in the ovary that is filled with old blood, also known as a "chocolate cyst". It occurs when endometriosis invades an ovary.

Endometriosis

A disease wherein the lining of the womb is displaced to other parts of the body such as ovaries fallopian tubes and peritoneum.

Endometritis

An inflammation or irritation of the lining of the uterus (the endometrium). It is not the same as endometriosis. It is typically caused by infections such as chlamydia, gonorrhea, tuberculosis, or mixtures of normal vaginal bacteria and is more likely to occur after miscarriage or childbirth, especially after a long labor or caesarian section.

Endometrium

The lining of the uterus which grows and sheds in response to estrogen and progesterone stimulation; the bed of tissue designed to nourish the implanted embryo.

Endorphins

Natural narcotics manufactured in the brain to reduce sensitivity to pain and stress. May contribute to stress-related fertility problems.

Endoscopy

The visualization of the internal organs and cavities of the body with illuminated optic instruments such as a laparoscope.

Endothelial cells

Simple cells forming the lining of all blood vessels and lymphatics.

Epigenetic

The study of changes in organisms caused by modification of gene expression rather than alteration of the genetic code itself.

Estrogen

The primary female hormone produced mainly by the ovaries.

Estradiol/Estrogen

The female sex hormone produced in the ovary. Its production is signaled by the pituitary gland in the brain and is responsible for formation of the female secondary sex characteristics. It supports the growth of the follicle and the development of the uterine lining. At midcycle the peak estrogen level triggers the release of the LH spike from the pituitary gland. The LH spike is necessary for the release of the ovum from the follicle. Fat cells can also produce estrogen, and this is known as aromatase.

Estrogen Replacement Therapy

Also referred to as Hormone Replacement Therapy (HRT). The practice of medically administering estrogen after the menopause, after procedures such as hysterectomy, or together with menopause-inducing drugs to reduce side effects and reduce medical risks such as osteoporosis.

Etiology

The study of all factors that may be involved in the development of a disease, the cause of a disease.

Expectant management

A "wait and see" approach, which involves no active intervention or treatment. The patient is followed closely to determine if any future action is needed.

Excision

A method of removing endometriosis by physically cutting it out of the body, normally via laparoscopy.

F

Fallopian tubes
Ducts through which eggs travel to the uterus once released from the ovary.

Fascia
Connective tissue supporting organ structures. Consisting of mostly collagen fibers, this tissue makes up ligaments and keeps muscular bundles together as well as lending structural integrity and strength to the body.

Fecundity
Ability to reproduce.

Fertility
The capacity to initiate or support conception.

Fertility treatment
Any method or procedure used to enhance fertility or increase the likelihood of pregnancy. The goal of fertility treatment is to help couples have a child.

Fertilization
The combining of the genetic material carried by sperm and egg to create an embryo. It normally occurs inside the fallopian tube (*in vivo*) but may also occur in a petri dish (*in vitro*). See also In Vitro Fertilization (IVF).

Fetus
A term used to refer to a baby during the period of gestation between eight weeks and term.

Fibroid (myoma or leiomyoma)
A benign tumor of the uterine muscle and connective tissue.

202 | GLOSSARY

Fimbria

The opening of the fallopian tube near the ovary. When stimulated by the follicular fluid released during ovulation, the fingerlike ends grasp the ovary and coax the egg into the tube.

Flare effect:

When taking GnRH agonists an increase in hormones occurs usually from four to ten days, causing a possible increase in symptoms in the first week or two of treatment.

Follicles

Fluid-filled sacs in the ovary which contain the eggs released at ovulation. Each month an egg develops inside the ovary in a fluid filled pocket called a follicle.

Follicular fluid

The fluid inside the follicle that cushions and nourishes the ovum. When released during ovulation, the fluid stimulates the fimbria to grasp the ovary and coax the egg into the fallopian tube.

Follicle Stimulating Hormone – FSH

A pituitary hormone that stimulates spermatogenesis and follicular development. In the man FSH stimulates the Sertoli cells in the testicles and supports sperm production. In the woman FSH stimulates the growth of the ovarian follicle. Elevated FSH levels are indicative of gonadal failure in both men and woman.

Follicular phase

The pre-ovulatory portion of a woman's cycle during which a follicle grows, and high levels of estrogen cause the lining of the uterus to proliferate (thicken). This normally takes between 12 and 14 days.

Fulguration

The surgical burning of tissue with modalities such as electrocautery.

G

Gamete
A reproductive cell: Sperm in men, the egg in women.

Gastrointestinal
Relating to the stomach and intestine.

Genitals
The external sex organs: the labia and clitoris in the woman, and the penis and the testicles in the man. Also called genitalia.

Genitourinary
Related to the genital and urinary systems of the body.

Genomics
The science that deals with the analysis of DNA (gene activity and expression) in body tissues and fluids with respect to specific diseases.

Germ cell
In the male the testicular cell that divides to produce the immature sperm cells; in the woman the ovarian cell that divides to form the egg (ovum). The male germ cell remains intact throughout the man's reproductive life; the woman uses up her germ cells at the rate of about one thousand per menstrual cycle, although usually only one egg matures each cycle.

GnRH analogue – gonadotrophin releasing hormone analogue
A class of drugs that are used to prevent the ovaries from releasing eggs too early during an IVF cycle. There are two types of GnRH analogues: GnRH agonists, which cause a sharp increase of LH and FSH, and GnRH antagonists, which cause immediate suppression of LH (= no "flare-up"). GnRH-analogues are also used to suppress ovarian function in women with endometriosis so that they do not menstruate, known as a medically induced menopause.

Gonadotropins

Hormones which control reproductive function: Follicle Stimulating Hormone and Luteinizing Hormone.

Gonadotropin Releasing Hormone – GnRH

A substance secreted by the hypothalamus every ninety minutes or so. This hormone enables the pituitary to secrete LH and FSH, which stimulate the gonads. See also FSH, LH.

Gonad

The gland that makes reproductive cells and "sex" hormones, such as the testicles, which make sperm and testosterone, and the ovaries, which produce eggs (ova) and estrogen.

H

Hematoma

Blood clot.

Hemoperitoneum

Escape of blood in the peritoneal cavity.

Hemorrhagic

Pertaining to bleeding from the blood vessels.

Hemostasis

The arrest of bleeding.

Hirsutism

Excessive body hair, such as a mustache or pubic hair growing upward toward the navel, found in women with excess androgens.

Hormone

A chemical secreted from a part of the body (usually an endocrine gland) and carried in the bloodstream to another part to stimulate or retard its function.

Hormone Replacement Therapy – HRT

Also referred to as Estrogen Replacement Therapy. The practice of medically administering estrogen after the menopause, after procedures such as hysterectomy, or together with menopause-inducing drugs to reduce side effects and reduce medical risks such as osteoporosis.

Human Chorionic Gonadotropin – hCG

The hormone produced in early pregnancy which keeps the corpus luteum producing progesterone. Also used via injection to trigger ovulation after some fertility treatments and used in men to stimulate testosterone production.

Human Menopausal Gonadotropin – hMG

A combination of the hormones FSH and LH, which is extracted from the urine of post-menopausal women. Used to induce ovulation in several fertility treatments.

Hyperplasia

Overgrowth of endometrial tissue that may sometimes be a precancerous condition.

Hyperprolactinemia

A condition in which the pituitary gland secretes too much prolactin. Prolactin can suppress LH and FSH production, reduce sex drive in the man, and directly suppress ovarian function in the woman.

Hyperstimulation – Ovarian Hyperstimulation Syndrome

A potentially life-threatening side effect of ovulation induction treatment. Arises when too many follicles develop and hCG is given to release the eggs. This may be prevented by withholding the hCG injection when ultrasound monitoring indicates that too many follicles have matured.

Hyperthyroidism

Overproduction of thyroid hormone by the thyroid gland. The resulting increased metabolism "burns up" estrogen too rapidly and interferes with ovulation.

Hypo estrogenic

Having lower than normal levels of estrogen.

Hypogonadotropic hypopituitarism

A spectrum of diseases resulting in low pituitary gland output of LH and FSH. Men with this disorder have low sperm counts and may lose their virility; women do not ovulate and may lose their secondary sex characteristics. Low sperm production.

Hypothalamus

A part of the brain, the hormonal regulation center, located adjacent to and above the pituitary gland. In both the man and the woman this tissue secretes GnRH every ninety minutes or so. The pulsatile GnRH enables the pituitary gland to secrete LH and FSH, which stimulate the gonads.

Hypothyroidism

A condition in which the thyroid gland produces an insufficient amount of thyroid hormone. The resulting lowered metabolism interferes with the normal breakdown of "old" hormones and causes lethargy. Men will suffer from a lower sex drive and elevated prolactin (see Hyperprolactinemia), and women will suffer from elevated prolactin and estrogen, both of which will interfere with fertility.

Hysterectomy

Surgical removal of the uterus. When the ovaries and the fallopian tubes are also removed, it is called hysterectomy with bilateral salpingo-oopherectomy. See also our article on <u>hysterectomy</u>.

Hysterosalpingogram (HSG)

An x-ray of the pelvic organs in which a radio-opaque dye is injected through the cervix into the uterus and fallopian tubes. This test checks for malformations of the uterus and blockage of the fallopian tubes.

Hysteroscopy

A procedure in which the doctor checks for uterine abnormalities by inserting a fiber-optic device. Minor surgical repairs can be executed during the procedure.

I

Implantation

The embedding of the embryo into tissue so it can establish contact with the mother's blood supply for nourishment. Implantation usually occurs in the lining of the uterus; however, in an ectopic pregnancy it may occur elsewhere in the body.

Immune system

The system within the body that secures against harmful substances; it enables the body to recognize materials as foreign to itself and to neutralize, eliminate, or metabolize them with or without injure to its own tissues.

Incidence

New occurrences of a disorder per year.

Inflammation

A tissue reaction to irritation, injury or infection, marked by localized warmth, swelling, redness and pain.

208 | GLOSSARY

Informed consent

A contractual agreement between a patient and a physician, whereby the patient gives permission to undergo a certain procedure based on as clear an understanding of the issue as is possible. This understanding should be based on information on and explanation of the procedure and the options available to the patient.

Intra-abdominal

Inside the abdominal cavity.

In Vitro Fertilization (IVF)

Literally means "in glass." Fertilization of an egg by sperm takes place outside the body in a small glass dish.

Infertility

The inability to conceive after a year of unprotected intercourse or the inability to carry a pregnancy to term.

Inhibin

A male feedback hormone made in the testicles to regulate FSH production by the pituitary gland.

Inhibin-F (Folliculostatin)

A female feedback hormone made in the ovary to regulate FSH production by the pituitary gland.

Intracrinology

The study of hormones that act inside a cell.

Intramuscular injection

A shot that is inserted into the muscle. Some IVF drugs are administered in the muscle, usually in the upper hip.

IUD (Intrauterine Device)

A device placed into the uterus to prevent pregnancy.

Intrauterine insemination (IUI)

A technique in which sperm are introduced directly into a woman's cervix or uterus to produce pregnancy, with or without ovarian stimulation to produce multiple eggs.

K

Karyotyping

A test performed to analyze chromosomes for the presence of genetic defects.

L

Laparoscope

The instrument used to perform a laparoscopy. It is a small telescope which can be inserted into a hole in the abdominal wall for viewing the internal organs.

Laparoscopy

A surgical procedure used as the primary means of diagnosing endometriosis; also used to treat endometriosis. A lighted tube is inserted into the belly button through which the surgeon can view the inside of the abdomen. Instruments can be inserted into other small incisions to remove or destroy endometriosis.

Laparotomy

Open abdominal surgery.

Laser

An extremely concentrated beam of light that can be directed precisely to destroy diseased tissue.

Laser ablation

A method of destroying endometriosis using a concentrated beam of light.

Laser surgery

Surgery that involves the utilization of a radiated light (laser) beam.

Leiomyoma

See Fibroids

Ligaments

Series of structures supporting the internal female genitalia within the pelvis. Ligaments associated with the female reproductive tract are the "broad", the "uterine", and the "ovarian".

Live birth rate

The rate of live births per cycle. Also known as "take home rate."

Lupus (systemic lupus erythematosus)

An inflammatory disease, generally occurring in young women which causes deterioration of the connective tissue and may attack soft internal organs as well as bones and muscles. Symptoms vary widely but may include fever rash, abdominal pains, weakness, fatigue and pains in joints and muscles.

Luteinizing Hormone (LH)

A pituitary hormone that stimulates the gonads. In the man LH is necessary for spermatogenesis (Sertoli cell function) and for the production of testosterone (Leydig cell function). In the woman LH is necessary for the production of estrogen. When estrogen reaches a critical peak, the pituitary releases a surge of LH (the LH spike), which releases the egg from the follicle.

LH Surge

The release of luteinizing hormone (LH) that causes the release of a mature egg from the follicle. Ovulation test kits detect the sudden increase of LH, signaling that ovulation is about to occur (usually within 24-36 hours).

Luteal phase

Post-ovulatory phase of a woman's cycle. The corpus luteum produces progesterone, which cause the uterine lining to thicken to support the implantation and growth of the embryo.

Luteal Phase Defect (LPD)

A condition that occurs when the uterine lining does not develop adequately because of inadequate progesterone stimulation, or because of the inability of the uterine lining to respond to progesterone stimulation. LPD may prevent embryonic implantation or cause an early miscarriage.

Luteinized Unruptured Follicle (LUF) syndrome

A condition in which the follicle develops and changes into the corpus luteum without releasing the egg.

M

Machine Learning

A branch of artificial intelligence in which a computer generates rules underlying or based on raw data that has been fed into it.

Macrophages

Immune cells that gobble up invaders.

Malignant

Cancerous, particularly when used to refer to a tumor or mass.

Menopause

The transition between the reproductive and post reproductive stages in an older women's life, or when a woman ceases to menstruate or ovulate.

Menorrhagia

Heavy or prolonged menstrual flow.

Menstruation

The physiologic cyclical shedding of the uterine endometrium (the lining of the uterus), unless pregnancy intervenes, and is characterized by vaginal bleeding of three to seven days' duration. Menstruation is also referred to as the "menstrual period" or "monthly period".

Metabolism

The sum of all the physical and chemical processes by which living organized substance is produced and maintained.

Metastasized

Refers to the spread of cancer

Metrorrhagia

Menstrual spotting during the middle of the cycle.

Microbiome

Microorganism that typically inhabit a particular environment such a site on or in an organism.

Microbiota

Microorganisms that typically inhabit a particular environment such site on or in an organism.

Miscarriage

Spontaneous loss of an embryo or fetus from the womb.

Mittelschmerz

Pain in the lower abdomen at the time of ovulation.

Modalities

Treatment application methods.

Morbidity

A diseased state/character, or ill health. Within a population it refers to the number of sick persons or cases of disease recorded.

Mortality

Death

Mucosa

Epithelial tissue encountered in the mouth, vagina, anus, etc.

Müllerian ducts

Ducts in the embryo that develops into the ovaries, uterus, and vagina.

Multiple pregnancies

A pregnancy that involves more than one fetus. For example, twins, triplets, and quadruplets are all multiple pregnancies. Multiple pregnancies are a risk associated with IVF.

Myofascial pain

An often-chronic condition affecting the fascia (connective tissue which covers the muscles), which may involve either a single muscle or whole muscle group. The area where pain is experienced may not be where the pain generator is located (known as "referred pain").

Myoma

See Fibroids.

Myomectomy

Surgery performed to remove fibroid tumors.

Myometrium

The middle, muscular layer of the uterus (which is what is affected if you have adenomyosis).

N

Nanomedicine

The branch of medicine concerned with the use of nanotechnology. Various types of nanoparticles re being used in nanomedicine especially, to diagnose and treat certain disorders.

Nanoparticle

Any of various microscopic particles especially, a single molecule with dimensions in the nanometer range.

Nonsteroidal anti-inflammatory drugs (NSAIDs)

Pain medication that works by inhibiting prostaglandins and that include ibuprofen, naproxen sodium and ketorolac tromethamine.

O

Oligomenorrhea

Infrequent menstrual periods.

Omentum

A membranous double layer of fatty tissue that covers and supports the intestines and organs in the lower abdominal area.

Oncology

The branch of medicine concerned with the study of and treatment of cancer.

Oophorectomy

Surgical removal of one or both ovaries.

Oocyte

The egg; the reproductive cell from the ovary; the female gamete; the sex cell that contains the woman's genetic information.

Organic

Organic foods are grown without the use of chemical pesticides and fertilizers, genetically engineered ingredients, or sewage sludge.

Osteoporosis

A disease of the bones in which the bones become thin and porous.

Ovarian Hyperstimulation Syndrome

A potentially life-threatening side effect of ovulation induction treatment. Arises when too many follicles develop and hCG is given to release the eggs. This may be prevented by withholding the hCG injection when ultrasound monitoring indicates that too many follicles have matured.

Ovaries

Two small organs on either side of a woman's lower pelvis which produce ova, or eggs, and hormones; the female gamete-producing glands.

Ovarian cyst

A fluid-filled sac inside the ovary. An ovarian cyst may be found in conjunction with ovulation disorders, tumors of the ovary, and endometriosis. See also endometrioma.

Ovarian failure

The failure of the ovary to respond to FSH stimulation from the pituitary because of damage to or malformation of the ovary. Diagnosed by elevated FSH in the blood.

Ovarian follicle

The ovum together with its surrounding cells, located within the ovary.

Ovulation

The cyclical occurrence in a woman's reproductive years when an egg is released from the ovary and picked up by the fallopian tubes and guided into the uterus where it will either be fertilized or discarded with menstruation.

Ovulation induction
Medical treatment performed to initiate ovulation.

Ovulation predictor test
A home test kit that help women detect the "LH surge" in their urine. A surge in the level of Luteinizing Hormone (LH) causes ovulation.

Ovulatory Failure (anovulation)
The failure to ovulate.

Ovum/ova
An egg(s).

P

PCBs (polychlorinated biphenyls)
A group of nonflammable chemicals that were widely used as coolants in electrical transformers, industrial lubricants, hydraulic fluids and in carbonless paper from 1929 until they were banned in 1978. Some PCBs persist in the environment for more than 100 years.

Panhypopituitarism
Complete pituitary gland failure.

Pap smear
A screening test for pre-cancerous changes of the uterine cervix.

Parity
Number of babies where the gestation went to term.

Patent

The condition of being open, as with the Fallopian tubes that form part of the reproductive organs.

Pelvic ultrasound

A procedure in which the doctor checks for structural abnormalities or other problems in the female reproductive system.

Pelvic Inflammatory Disease (PID)

An infection in the pelvic area that can be caused by a variety of bacteria and can attack various pelvic organs.

Perimetrium

The outer lining, layer/muscular coat of the uterus.

Perineal body

The thickened part between the anal and vaginal openings.

Peritoneum

A smooth membrane lining the walls of the abdominal and pelvic cavities and enclosing the organs.

PGD

Pre-implantation genetic diagnosis: a diagnostic technique involving genetic tests on an embryo. Generally done when the embryo is at the six to eight cell stage when one cell is removed for analysis of its DNA or chromosomes to determine whether or not the embryo is like to develop a genetic disease.

PGS

Pre-implantation genetic screening: using genetic techniques to check if an embryo has the right number of chromosomes. Although used particularly for older women (at increased risk of chromosomal abnormalities) and for women who have had recurrent miscarriage (often due to

218 | GLOSSARY

chromosomal abnormalities), it is still in the experimental phase, since it is not yet evidence based.

Pituitary gland

The master gland; the gland that is stimulated by the hypothalamus and controls all hormonal functions. Located at the base of the brain just below the hypothalamus, this gland controls many major hormonal factories throughout the body including the gonads, the adrenal glands, and the thyroid gland.

Phthalates

Chemical compounds in plastics. Some have estrogenic activity, additionally some are cancer-causing.

Phytoestrogens

Weak, naturally occurring estrogenic compounds found in some plants such as flaxseed and soybeans.

Phytoremediation

The use of plants and trees to remove or neutralize contaminants.

Placenta

The embryonic tissue that invades the uterine wall and provides a mechanism for exchanging the baby's waste products for the mother's nutrients and oxygen. The baby is connected to the placenta by the umbilical cord.

Pneumothorax

Air leaks into the space between the lungs and chest wall.

Polycystic Ovarian Syndrome (PCOS)

A condition found in women who don't ovulate, characterized by excessive production of androgens (male sex hormones) and the presence of cysts in the ovaries. Though PCOS can be without symptoms, some include excessive weight gain, acne, and excessive hair growth.

Posterior
Bottom or lower.

Postpartum
After delivery. This period lasts until six weeks after delivery.

Pre-embryo
The fertilized egg that is produced outside the uterus during IVF.

Premature menopause
Menopause that occurs naturally before the age of 40. Also known as premature ovarian failure.

Premature ovarian failure
A condition where the ovary runs out of follicles before the normal age associated with menopause.

Presacral neurectomy
A surgical procedure in which nerves at the back of the uterus are severed in an attempt to eliminate or reduce pain.

Prevalence
Occurrence of a disorder in the general population.

Primary Dysmenorrhea
Painful periods and other symptoms in the absence of pelvic pathology.

Primary infertility
Infertility in a woman who has never had a pregnancy.

Progesterone
The hormone produced by the corpus luteum during the second half of a woman's cycle. It thickens the lining of the uterus to prepare it to accept implantation of a fertilized egg.

Prognosis
Prediction of most likely future outcome.

Prolactin
The hormone that stimulates the production of milk in breastfeeding women..

Prostaglandins
Substances found in bodily tissues which are often responsible for the contractions of smooth muscles such as the uterus. Prostaglandins keep blood pressure low and influence hormone activity.

Proteomics
The science that deals with the analysis of proteins (presence, activity, function, dysfunction) in body tissues and fluids with respect to specific diseases.

Puberty
The time of life when the body begins making adult levels of sex hormones (estrogen or testosterone) and the youngster takes on adult body characteristics: developing breasts, growing a beard, pubic hair, and auxiliary hair; attaining sexual maturity.

R

Recurrent miscarriage
Three or more miscarriages. Also know as recurrent pregnancy loss.

Recto-vaginal septum
The fascial layer which separates the vagina from the rectum.

Resection
Surgical excision (removal by cutting) of a portion of an organ or other structure.

ENDOMETRIOSIS | 221

Resistant ovary

An ovary that cannot respond to the follicle-stimulating message sent by FSH. Primitive germ cells will be present in the ovary; however, they will not respond to FSH stimulation.

Retroverted Uterus

Tilted uterus.

Ruptured ectopic pregnancy

Ectopic pregnancy that has eroded or torn through the tissue in which it has implanted, producing hemorrhage (bleeding) from exposed vessels.

S

Sacroiliac

Joint in lower back where the spine meets the pelvis. A number of conditions, including <u>endometriosis</u>, may cause discomfort in this area.

Sacrospinous ligament

Ligament attaching the ischial spine to the sacrum.

Salpingectomy

Surgical removal of the fallopian tube.

Salpingitis

Inflammation of the Fallopian tube.

Salpingostomy/Fimbrioplasty

Surgical repair made to the fallopian tubes; a procedure used to open the fimbria.

Secondary Dysmenorrhea

Painful periods due to pelvic pathology or a recognized medical condition.

222 | GLOSSARY

Secondary infertility

The inability of a couple which has successfully achieved pregnancy to achieve another. In other words: it refers to a couple which has one biological child but is unable to conceive another.

Septate uterus

A uterus divided into right and left halves by a wall of tissue (septum). Women with a septate uterus have an increased chance of early pregnancy loss.

Sexually transmitted disease (STD)

An infection that is spread by sexual contact. Also called a sexually transmitted infection (STI).

Sjögren's Syndrome

An autoimmune disorder in which deficient moisture production can affect the eyes, salivary glands in the mouth and other mucous membranes. Abnormal dryness can lead to damage to the eyes, dental disorder, lungs, and other problems.

Sonogram (ultrasound)

Use of high-frequency sound waves for creating an image of internal body parts.

Spontaneous Abortion

Miscarriage.

Stem cell

A "blank" cell, capable of becoming another cell such as a skin cell, a muscle cell, or nerve cell.

Sterility

An irreversible condition that prevents conception.

Stillbirth
The death of a fetus between the twentieth week of gestation and birth.

Subcutaneous injection
A shot that is inserted under the skin, including the upper thigh, abdomen, or upper arm.

Superfund
The common name given to the law called the Comprehensive Environmental Response, Compensation and Liability Act of 1980 or CERCLA. Superfund is also the trust fund set up by Congress to handle emergency and hazardous waste sites needing long-term cleanup.

Superovulation
Stimulation of multiple ovulations with fertility drugs; also known as controlled ovarian hyperstimulation (COH).

Surgical Menopause
Menopause brought on by surgical removal of the ovaries,

T

T cells; T lymphocytes
Small white blood cells that orchestrate and/or directly participate in the immune defense they are processed in the thymus and secrete lymphokines.

Testosterone
The male hormone responsible for the formation of secondary sex characteristics and for supporting the sex drive. Testosterone is also necessary for spermatogenesis.

224 | GLOSSARY

Thoracoscopy

A procedure performed under general anesthesia that uses an instrument with a light source to look into the space inside of the chest, outside of the lungs.

Thromboembolisms

Blood clotting and migration of clots to plug distant blood vessels.

Thyroid conditions

Any condition in which the thyroid is not functioning properly, such as underactive (hypo) or overactive (hyper) thyroid.

Thyroid gland

The endocrine gland in the front of the neck that produces thyroid hormones to regulate the body's metabolism.

TNF

A molecule that is important in inflammation. TNF binding protein blocks the activity of TNF and selectively inhibits inflammation.

Transvaginal ultrasonography

Ultrasonography which sends into the pelvic cavity and receives ultrasonic waves through the vagina by using a probe placed inside the vagina.

Trimester

One-third of the length of a pregnancy (3 months).

Tubal ligation

A type of female sterilization in which the fallopian tubes are cut, clipped, or tied in order to prevent pregnancy.

Tubocornual anastomosis

Surgery performed to remove a blocked portion of the fallopian tube and to reconnect the tube to the uterus. Tubouterine implantation may also be performed to remove fallopian tube blockage near the uterus and reimplant the tube in the uterus.

Tubotubal anastomosis
Surgery performed to remove a diseased portion of the fallopian tube and reconnect the two ends; sterilization reversal.

Turner's Syndrome
The most common genetic defect contributing to female fertility problems. The ovaries fail to form and appear as slender threads of atrophic ovarian tissue, referred to as streak ovaries. Karyotyping will reveal that this woman has only one female (X) chromosome instead of two.

U

Ultrasound
A test used to visualize the reproductive organs. The instrument works by bouncing sound waves off the organs, and a picture displayed on a TV screen shows the internal organs.

Ultrasonography
The delineation of deep bodily structures by sending ultrasonic waves (sound waves of frequency higher than the range audible to the human ear, i.e.. above 20,000 cycles per second) toward an organ or mass, which in turn bounces back (echoes); the patterns produce are graphically displayed on a fluorescent screen for interpretation.

Umbilicus
The navel or belly button.

Umbilical cord
Two arteries and one vein encased in a gelatinous tube leading from the baby to the placenta. Used to exchange nutrients and oxygen from the mother for waste products from the baby.

226 | GLOSSARY

Unexplained infertility

Infertility for which the cause cannot be determined with currently available diagnostic techniques.

Unicornuate uterus

An abnormality in which the uterus is "one sided" and smaller than usual.

Ureter

The muscular tubes carrying urine from the kidneys to the bladder.

Urethra

The tube that allows urine to pass between the bladder and the outside of the body.

Urinary tract disorders

Disorders of the urinary tract causing painful urination, frequency of urination, and/or urine leakage, such as interstitial cystitis. Sometimes confused with the symptoms of endometriosis on the bladder.

Uterine fibroids

Abnormal, benign (non-cancerous) growths of muscle within the wall of a woman's uterus.

Uterine polyps

Abnormal, benign (non-cancerous) growths attached to a short stalk that protrudes from the inner surface of a woman's uterus.

Uterosacral ligament

Ligaments attaching the lower part of the uterus to the sacral bone. One of the main supports of the uterus and upper vagina, and a common place to find endometriosis.

Uterus

The hollow, muscular organ that houses and nourishes the fetus during pregnancy.

V

Vagina
The canal leading from the cervix to the outside of the woman's body; the birth passage.

Vaginismus
Painful spasm of pelvic floor muscles on vaginal entry, such as sexual intercourse.

Vaginitis
Clinical inflammation of the vagina.

Vaporization
A method of destroying endometriosis by boiling of the cellular water with a laser or electrosurgical knife.

Venereal Disease
Any infection that can be sexually transmitted, such as chlamydia, gonorrhea, ureaplasma, and syphilis.

Venous
Having, characterized by, or composed of veins, the vessels of the body that return blood from arms, legs and organs back to the heart.

Vulva
The female external genital organs.

Vulvodynia
Painful vulva, also sometimes associated with urinary symptoms, painful intercourse and generalized pelvic pain.

X

X chromosome

The congenital, developmental, or genetic information in the cell that transmits the information necessary to make a female. All eggs contain one X chromosome, and half of all sperm carry an X chromosome. When two X chromosomes combine, the baby will be a girl. See also Y chromosome.

Y

Y chromosome

The genetic material that transmits the information necessary to make a male. The Y chromosome can be found in one-half of the man's sperm cells. When an X and a Y chromosome combine, the baby will be a boy. See also X Chromosome.

Z

Zona pellucida

The outer protein coat (shell) of an ovum, which must be penetrated by a sperm cell for fertilization to take place.

Zygote

A fertilized egg which has not yet divided.

RESOURCES

The following is a list of resources that may prove useful.

The Endometriosis Association is the premier endometriosis organization founded by Mary Lou Ballweg in 1980, whose mission is to find a cure and prevention for endometriosis while at the same time providing education, support, and research to those affected. The organization runs support groups; publishes educational material such as brochures, books, and supports research:

Endometriosis Association International Headquarters
8585 North 76th Place
Milwaukee, WI 53223 USA
Phone: 1.414.355.2200
Toll Free: 1.800.992.3636
Fax: 1.414.355.6065
Email:support@endometriosisassn.org
Website: endometriosisassn.org

The Endometriosis Foundation of America (EndoFound) strives to increase disease recognition, provide advocacy, facilitate expert surgical training, and fund landmark endometriosis research.

230 | RESOURCES

Engaged in a robust campaign to inform both the medical community and the public, the EndoFound places particular emphasis on the critical importance of early diagnosis and effective intervention while simultaneously providing education to the next generation of medical professionals and their patients.\

Endometriosis Foundation of America

872 Fifth Avenue New York, NY 10065
Phone: 212-988-4160
Website: www.endofound.org

Endometriosis.org is the global platform which links all stake holders in endometriosis - one of the most common causes of pelvic pain and infertility in women. The organization provides current information and news about endometriosis. This knowledge empowers those with endometriosis to make informed decisions about their treatment options.

Website: endometriosis.org

The Endometriosis Research Center (ERC) was founded in early 1997 by Executive Director Michelle Marvel with the vision of addressing the ongoing need for international endometriosis awareness, advocacy, support, education, legislative efforts and research facilitation. Since the founding, the organization has been giving a voice to those with the disease.

Endometriosis Research Center
630 Ibis Drive
Delray Beach, FL 33444

E-mail: askerc@endocenter.org

Toll Free: (800) 239-7280

Fax: (561) 274-09

Other entities and sources of information

The American Association of Gynecologic Laparoscopists
www.aagl.org

The American College of Obstetrics and Gynecologists
www.acog.org

The American Society for Reproductive Medicine
www.asrm.org

The Office of Women's Health
www.womenshealth.gov

World Endometriosis Society
www.endometriosis.ca

The World Health Organization
www.who.int

United States Environmental Protection Agency
https://www.epa.gov/superfund

AirNow.gov - Home of the U.S. Air Quality Index
https://www.airnow.gov

SYMPTOMS TRACKER

Menstrual Symptoms Tracker

Keep track of the symptoms you experience throughout your entire menstrual cycle. Mark which symptoms, if any, you experience each day. For a more detailed record, include a rank 1-5 based on how severe you experience each symptom in a day. Share this tracker with your gynecologist to help explain your pain and period symptoms.

Month_____

	1	2	3	4	5	6	7	8	9	10	11	12	13	14	15	16	17	18	19	20	21	22	23	24	25	26	27	28	29	30	31
Heavy bleeding																															
Moderate bleeding																															
Light bleeding																															
Spotting																															
Severe cramps																															
Moderate cramps																															
Light cramps																															
Painful sex																															
Nausea																															
Diarrhea																															
Painful defecation																															
Back pain																															
Leg pain																															

REFERENCES

CHAPTER I

Introduction

1. Cook, A, Stop Endometriosis and Pelvic Pain, Femsana Press, Los Gatos, CA 2012

2. Ballweg, M.L., Overcoming endometriosis, new help from the endometriosis association, Endometriosis Association, Lincolnwood,1987

3. Seckin, T, Diagnosing Endometriosis, https://drseckin.com/ June 10, 2020

4. Agarwal, SK, Chapron, C, Giuice, LC, Missmer, SA, Singh, SS, Taylor, HS, Clinical Diagnosis of Endometriosis: a call to action, AJOG, vol 220 issue 4

5. Acién, P, Velasco, I, Endometriosis: A Disease That Remains Enigmatic, Obstetrics and Gynecology, Volume 2013,

6. Brosens, I, Benagiano, G, Endometriosis, a modern syndrome, Indian J Med Res. 2011 Jun; 133(6): 581–593.

7. Novak, ER, and Woodruff, JD, Novak's Gynecologic and Obstetrical Pathology, WB Saunders, Philadelphia, 1979

8. Nezhat C, Nezhat F, Nezhat C: Endometriosis: ancient disease, ancient treatments. Fertil Steril 2012;98(suppl 6):S1-S62

236 | REFERENCES

9. Mandal, A, Laparoscopic Surgery History, News Medical Life Sciences, Nov 2022, https://www.news-medical.net/medical/authors/ananya-mandal

10. Benagiano G, Brosens I: Who identified endometriosis? Fertil Steril 2011;95:13-16.

11. Audebert A, Backstrom T, Barlow DH, et al: Endometriosis 1991: a discussion document. Hum Reprod 1992;7:432-435

CHAPTER II
Theories on the Cause of Endometriosis

1. https://www.endofound.org/what-causes-endometriosis

2. https://www.who.int/news-room/fact-sheets/detail/endometriosis

3. Sampson, JA (1927). Metastatic or embolic endometriosis, due to the menstrual dissemination of endometrial tissue into the venous circulation. *The American Journal of Pathology, 3*(2): 93–110.143.

4. https://drseckin.com/is-endometriosis-genetic/?gclid=CjwKCAjwk-MeUBhBuEiwA4hpqEH7hmBPGBzpYNaikRNXcXTtCkiuOkTLBvaIXGKw1RzM07AH8TDpOEBoCEiEQAvD_BwE

5 https://www.endonews.com/an-important-environmental-contaminant-dioxin-has-links-to-the-pathogenesis-of-endometriosis

6. Carpinello, O, Sundheimer, L, Alford, C Endometriosis Last Update: October 22, 2017

7. Genetic, Epigenetic, and Steroidogenic Modulation Mechanisms in Endometriosis *J. Clin. Med.* 2020, *9*(5), 309; https://doi.org/10.3390/jcm9051309

8. Sun-Wei Guo, Sun-Wei, Epigenetics of endometriosis Molecular Human Reproduction, Vol.15, No.10 pp. 587–607, 2009

9. Hsiao K-Y, Wu M-H, Tsai S-J. Epigenetic regulation of the pathological process in endometriosis. Reprod Med Biol. 2017;16:314-319. https://doi.org/10.1002/rmb2.12047

10. https://www.glowm.com/sectionview/heading/Genetics%20of%20Endometriosis/item/362#.YpMEtS2z0_U

11. Harada,T, Endometriosis pathogenesis and treatment, Springer, Japan 201412. Sourial, S, Tempest, N, Hapangama, D, Theories on the Pathogenesis of Endometriosis, Int J Reprod Med. 2014; 2014: 179515.

13. Burney RO, Giudice L. Pathogenesis and pathophysiology of endometriosis. *Fertility and Sterility*. 2012;98:511–519.

14. Giudice LC Endometriosis. *The New England Journal of Medicine*. 2010;362(25):2389–2398.

15. Acién P, Velasco, I, Endometriosis: A Disease That Remains Enigmatic, Volume 2013 | Article ID 242149

CHAPTER III

Environmental Toxins and Endometriosis

1. Ballweg, ML., Endometriosis, the complete reference for taking charge of your health, Contemporary Books, Chicago 2004

2 https://ejatlas.org/conflict/mossville-louisiana-environmental-racism-united-states

3 https://www.washingtonpost.com/climate-environment/2020/08/28/hurricane-laura-chemicals-pollution/

238 | REFERENCES

4 https://www.theguardian.com/us-news/2021/nov/17/this-communitys-black-families-lost-their-ancestral-homes-their-white-neighbors-got-richer

5 https://theintercept.com/2015/11/04/erasing-mossville-how-pollution-killed-a-louisiana-town/
https://news.un.org/en/story/2021/03/1086172

6 https://www.blackpast.org/african-american-history/cancer-alley-louisiana-1987/

7 https://meannow.wordpress.com/life-in-mossville/

8 Helm, J, Nishioka, M, Brody, J, Rudel, R, Dobson, R Measurement of endocrine disrupting and asthma-associated chemicals in hair products used by black women, Journal Environmental Research 2018

9 Black Women for Wellness www.bwwla.com • www.bwwla.org

10. Zota, A, Shamasunder, B, The environmental injustice of beauty: framing chemical exposures from beauty products as a health disparities concern

10 The environmental injustice of beauty: framing chemical exposures from beauty products as a health disparities concern Ami R Zota, ScD, MS; Bhavna Shamasunder, PhD, MES

11. Cook, A, Stop Endometriosis and Pelvic Pain, Femsana Press, Los Angeles, CA, 2012

12.https://www.trinityschool.org/blog/?pid=71&p=&gclid=Cj0KCQiA09eQBhCxARIsAAYRiylTpGO KKtjNLHEBtKJp-BUcCtNu9UMqz9cZFnLoVnOInR6mv6-bmJc4aAqcJEALw_wcB

13. https://www.webmd.com/diet/ss/slideshow-best-worst-fish

14. https://www.healthline.com/health/food-nutrition/11-best-fish-to-eat
15. https://www.cleanwateraction.org/2020/07/29/bottled-water-human-health-consequences-drinking-plastic
16. https://culligankansascity.com/what-are-the-benefits-of-drinking-filtered-water/
17. https://www.respira.ca/blogs/news/phytoremediation-for-home-health?customer_posted=true#footer-newsletters
18.https://www.activebeat.com/your-health/8-houseplants-that-clean-and-promote-air-quality/3/
19. Pourzamani, T, Hajizadeh, Y Chemosphere. 2018 Apr;197:375-381.
20. Burchett, W, Orwell, RA, Torpy, T Plant/soil capacities to remove harmful substances from polluted indoor air. Plants and environmental quality group, (2002), Centre for Ecotoxicology, UTS, Australia (Bezugsquelle: www.plants-for-people.de
21. Bilthoven, NL, World Health Organization (WHO), (2000) The right to healthy indoor air—report on a WHO meeting, European Health Targets 10, 13
22. https://www.healthline.com/health/taking-off-your-shoes
23 https://environmentalpaper.org/wp-content/uploads/2018/03/RL_7mars_2018-1.pdf
24. https://www.thisoldhouse.com/cleaning/22759439/diy-natural-cleaning-products
25. https://thelistwire.usatoday.com/lists/5-reasons-to-use-safe-natural-cleaning-products/
26. https://www.webmd.com/allergies/hepa-filters-for-allergies

240 | REFERENCES

27. https://www.epa.gov/sites/default/files/201405/documents/healthy_homes_brochure_english.pdf
28. Bullard, R, Mohai, P, Saha, R, Wright, B, Toxic Wastes and Race at Twenty 1987—2007A Report Prepared for the United Church of Christ Justice & Witness Ministries, United Church of Christ © March 2007

CHAPTER IV

Pain and other symptoms

1. Carpinello, O, Endometriosis https://www.endotext.org/chapter/endometriosis/
2. HTTPS://WWW.WEBMD.COM/WOMEN/ENDOMETRIOSIS/UNDERSTANDING-ENDOMETRIOSIS-SYMPTOMS
3. HTTPS://EIGHTYSIXTHEENDO.COM/WHAT-IS-ENDOMETRIOSIS/
4. HTTPS://WWW.MYENDOMETRIOSISTEAM.COM/RESOURCES/SYMPTOMS-OF-ENDOMETRIOSIS
5. HTTPS://WWW.HOPKINSMEDICINE.ORG/HEALTH/CONDITIONS-AND-DISEASES/ENDOMETRIOSIS
6. Signorile PG, Cassano M, Viceconte R, Marcattilj V, Baldi A. Endometriosis: A Retrospective Analysis of Clinical Data from a Cohort of 4,083 Patients, With Focus on Symptoms. *In Vivo*. 2022;36(2):874-883. doi:10.21873/invivo.12776
7. Giudice, LC, Endometriosis, N Engl J Med 2010;362:2389-98.
8. Carson, SA, Kallen, AN, Diagnosis and Management of Infertility A Review JAMA July 6, 2021 Volume 326, Number 1
9. Bulun, S, Mechanisms of Disease Endometriosis, N Engl J Med 2009;360:268-79.

10. Shigesi, N, et al. "The association between endometriosis and autoimmune diseases: a systematic review and meta-analysis." *Human reproduction update* vol. 25,4 (2019): 486-503. doi:10.1093/humupd/dmz014

11. HTTPS://WWW.MYENDOMETRIOSISTEAM.COM/RESOURCES/THE-CONNECTION-BETWEEN-ENDOMETRIOSIS-AND-FIBROMYALGIA

12. https://www.who.int/news-room/fact-sheets/detail/endometriosis

13. Abisror N, Kolanska K, Cheloufi M, Selleret L, d'Argent E, Kayem G, et al. Endometriosis and autoimmunity. Explor Immunol. 2022;2:25–31. https://doi.org/10.37349/ei.2022.00034

14. Yusuf, A, The Clinical Anatomy of Endometriosis: A Review 10.7759/ CUREUS, 2018

15. Zondervan, K.T., Becker, C.M., Missmer, S.A., Endometriosis, N Engl J Med 382;13 nejm.org March 26, 2020

16. ESHRE Endometriosis Guideline Development Group 2022 www.eshre.eu/guidelines European Society of Human Reproduction and Embryology Follow us! Guideline of European Society of Human Reproduction and Embryology

17. Gater et al. Journal of Patient-Reported Outcomes (2020) 4:13 https://doi.org/10.1186/s41687-020-0177-3 ARCH Development and content validation of two new patient-reported outcome measures for endometriosis: the Endometriosis Symptom Diary (ESD) and Endometriosis Impact Scale (EIS) 1* 2 3 3,4 3 Adam Gater , Fiona Taylor , Christian

18. Seitz , C, Kamonthip, G, Wichmann, C and Haberland, C, Journal of Patient- Reported Outcomes

CHAPTER V
Infertility and Endometriosis

1, Strathy, JH, Molgaard, A, Coulam, CB, Melton, LF, Endometriosis and infertility: a laparoscopic study of endometriosis among fertile and infertile women Sterility and Fertility Vol. 38 PP 667-672, December 1982

2. Endometriosis and infertility a committee opinion, Fertility and Sterility Vol. 98, No.3, September 2012

3. Schenken, R, Infertility Aspects of Endometriosis, *Glob. libr. women's med, (ISSN: 1756-2228)* 2008

4. Taylor, HS, Pal, L, Seli, E, Speroff's Clinical Gynecologic Endocrinology and Infertility, Wolters Kluwer, Philadelphia, 2020

5. Lessey, BA, Medical management of endometriosis and infertility FERTILITY AND STERILITY *VOL. 73, NO. 6, JUNE 2000*

6. Fitz, VW, Minis,., Petrozza, J. Look (more carefully) before you leap: systematic ultrasounds for endometriosis in patients with subfertility Fertility and Sterility, November 2022 Volume 118 Issue 5p813-998

7. Alson, S, Jokubkiene, L, Henic, E, Sladkevicius, P, Prevalence of endometrioma and deep infiltrating endometriosis at transvaginal ultrasound examination of subfertile women undergoing assisted reproductive treatment, Sterility and Fertility, November 2022, Vol.118, 1ssue 5

8. Hodgson, RM, Lee,L,Wang, R, Mol, BWJohnson, N Interventions for endometriosis-related infertility: a systematic review and network meta-analysis Fertility and Sterility® Vol. 113, No. 2, February 2020

9. Vercellini, P,Barbara, G,Somigliana, E, Which treatments are effective for endometriosis-related infertility? Sterility and Fertility VOL. 113 NO. 2 / FEBRUARY 2020
10. Pirtea, P, Vulliemoz, N, de Ziegler, D. Ayoubi, JM, Infertility workup: identifying endometriosis, Fertility and Sterility Vol. 118Issue May 11, 2022
11. Bulletti, C, Cocci, ME, Battistoni, S, Borini, A, Endometriosis and infertility, J Assist Reprod Genet. 2010 Aug; 27(8): 441–447.
12. Alimi, Y, Iwanaga, J, Loukas, M, Tubbs, S, The Clinical Anatomy of Endometriosis: A Review, Cureus. 2018 Sep

CHAPTER VI
Fibroid Tumors and Endometriosis

1. Fibroids, Hopkinsmedicine.org, https://www.hopkinsmedicine.org/health/conditions-and-diseases/uterine-fibroids
2. Uimari, O, Järvelä, L and Ryynänen, M, Do symptomatic endometriosis and uterine fibroids appear together? J Hum Reprod Sci. 2011 Jan-Apr;
3. Charifson, MA, Vieira, D, Shaw, J, Kehoe, S, and Quinn, GP, Why are Black individuals disproportionately burdened with uterine fibroids and how are we examining this disparity? A systematic review Fertil Steril Rev® Vol. 3, No. 4, October 2022
4. Huang JQ, Lathi RB, Lemyre M, Rodriquez HE, Nezhat CH, Nezhat C. Coexistence of endometriosis in women with symptomatic leiomyomas. *Fertil Steril.* 2010;94:720–3.

5. Stringer, NH, Uterine Fibroids, what every woman needs to know, Physicians and Scientist Publishing Co, Glenview, IL, 1996

6. Weather, L, endometriosis, fibroids and cyclic pelvic pain; AAGL. 1997

7. Al-Hendy, A, Lukes, S, Poindexter, AN, Venturella, R, Villarroel, C, Critchley, H, Treatment of Uterine Fibroid Symptoms with Relugolix Combination Therapy, February 18, 2021 N Engl J Med 2021;

8. Schlaff, WD, Ackerman, RT, Al-Hendy, A, Archer, DF, Barnhart, KT, Bradley, LD, Elagolix for Heavy Menstrual Bleeding in Women with Uterine Fibroids, January 23, 2020 N Engl J Med 2020

9. Simon, JA., Al-Hendy, A, Archer, DF. Barnhart, KT, Bradley, LD, Carr, BR, Elagolix Treatment for Up to 12 Months in Women With Heavy Menstrual Bleeding and Uterine Leiomyomas Obstetrics & Gynecology: June 2020 - Volume 135 - Issue 6 - p 1313-1326

10. Owens, C, The Diagnosis and Treatment of Endometriosis and Uterine Fibroids, Consultant360., September 20, 2021., https://www.consultant360.com/exclusive/obstetrics-gynecology/uterine-fibroids-excellence-forum/diagnosis-and-treatment

11. Weather, L, C02 Laser Myomectomy JNMA. vol 78, no. 10, 1986

12. Ivanova, Y, Dimitrov, D, Dimitrova, K, Shanker, A, Yordanov, A, The use of ultrasound guided high intensity focused ultrasound (HIFU) in the treatment of uterine fibroids, an overview, Wiad Lek 2022

13. Parker, PH, Uterine myomas: management, Fertility and Sterility Vol. 88, No. 2, August 2007

14. Taylor, HS, Pal, L, Seli, Clinical Gynecologic Endocrinology and Infertility, Wolters Kluwer, Philadelphia, 2020

15. AAGL Practice Report: Practice Guidelines for the Diagnosis and Management of Submucous Leiomyomas, Journal of Minimally Invasive Gynecology, Vol 19, No 2, March/April 2012

16. Johnson, TC, What Are the Treatments for Uterine Fibroids? WebMD November 10, 2020, https://www.webmd.com/women/uterine-fibroids/under-standing-uterine-fibroids-treatment

17. Stewart, EA, Uterine Fibroids, The Complete Guide, John Hopkins University Press, Baltimore, 2007

18. Goodwin, C, Broder, M, What Your Doctor May Not Tell You About Fibroids, Warner Books, New York, 2003

19. Fibroids, "An Essential Guide for the Newly Diagnosed," Johanna Skilling, Marlowe and Company, 2002, New York, NY

20. 2022 National Women's Health Network, Treating Fibroids and Endometriosis with Hormone-lowering Medications, Feb. 8, 2021, https://nwhn.org/treatingfibroids/ https://nwhn.org/treatingfibroids/

21. George AV, Allaire, C, Laberge, PY, Leyland, N, The Management of Uterine Leiomyomas, SOGC, Clinical Practice Guideline, No. 318, February 2015

22. Dixon, D, Parrott, EC, Segars, JH, Olden, K, and Pinn, VW, The Second NIH International Congress on Advances in Uterine Leiomyoma Research: Fertility and Sterility, Vol 86, No. 4, Oct. 2006

23. Chohan, L, Richardson, DL, Opportunistic Salpingectomy as a Strategy for Epithelial Ovarian Cancer Prevention, ACOG Committee on Gyn. Practice No. 774, Jan 2020

Chapter VII

Adenomyosis and Endometriosis

1. Stump-Sutiff, KA, Differences Between Endometriosis and Adenomyosis WebMD, September 02, 2022
   https://www.webmd.com/women/endometriosis/women-endometriosis-vs-adenomyosis

2. G. Leyendecker, G, Bilgicyildirim, A, Inacker, M, Stalf, T, Huppert, P, Adenomyosis and endometriosis. Re-visiting their association and further insights into the mechanisms of auto-traumatization. An MRI study, Arch Gynecol Obstet (2015) 291:917–932

3. Cope, AG, Khan, Z, VanBuren, WM, Green, IC, Burnett, TL, Concomitant endometriosis in patients undergoing hysterectomy with suspected adenomyosis Fertility and Sterility vol 114, iaauw 3 supplement E202, September 01, 2020 |

4. Almendrala, A, Adenomyosis vs. Endometriosis: What's the Difference? Health, June 25, 2022
   https://www.health.com/condition/endometriosis/adenomyosis-vs-endometriosis

5. Byrd, F, What Is Adenomyosis? WebMD, December 04, 2020,
   https://www.webmd.com/women/guide/adenomyosis-symptoms-causes-treatments

6. Maheshwari, A, Gurunath, S, Fatima, F, Bhattacharya, S,Adenomyosis and subfertility: a systematic review of prevalence, diagnosis, treatment and fertility outcomes *Human Reproduction Update*, Volume 18, Issue 4, July 2012, Pages 374–392,

7. Vannuccini, S, Luisi, S, Tosti, C, Sorbi, F, Petraglia, F, ,Role of medical therapy in the management of uterine adenomyosis Fertility and Sterility® Vol. 109, No. 3, March 2018

8. *Kimura, F, Takahashi, K, Takebayashi, K, Fujiwara, M,* Concomitant treatment of severe uterine adenomyosis in a premenopausal woman with an aromatase inhibitor and a gonadotropin-releasing hormone agonist Fertility and Sterility⊠ Vol. 87, No. 6, June 2007

9. Muneyyirci-Delale, O, Archer, DF, Owens, CD, Barnhart, KT, Bradley, LD, Efficacy and safety of elagolix with add-back therapy in women with uterine fibroids and coexisting adenomyosis Fertil Steril Rep® Vol. 2, No. 3, September 2021

10. Dessouky, R, Gamil, SA, Nada, MGR., and Libda, Y· Management of uterine adenomyosis: current trends and uterine artery embolization as a potential alternative to hysterectomy Insights Imaging. 2019 Dec; 10: 48.

11. Osada, H, Uterine adenomyosis and adenomyoma: the surgical approach, Fertility and Sterility® Vol. 109, No. 3, March 2018

12. Parker, JD, Leondires, M, Sinaii, N, Premkumar, A, Nieman, LK, Stratton,P., Persistence of dysmenorrhea and nonmenstrual pain after optimal endometriosis surgery may indicate adenomyosis Fertility and Sterility⊠ Vol. 86, No. 3, September 2006

13. Grimbizis GF, Mikos, T, Tarlatzis, B, Uterus-sparing operative treatment for adenomyosis Fertility and Sterility® Vol. 101, No. 2, February 2014

14. Givens, MB, Lindheim, SR, Goodman,LR, New approaches in bloom: four-petal adenomyomectomy technique Fertility and Sterility VOL. 114 NO. 6 / DECEMBER 2020

15. Bourdon, M, Santulli, P, Oliveira, J, Marcellin, L, Maignien, C, Melka, L, Focal adenomyosis is associated with primary infertility Fertil Steril! 2020;114:1271–7

16. Benagiano, G, Habiba, M, Brosens, I, The pathophysiology of uterine adenomyosis: an update Fertility and Sterility® Vol. 98, No. 3, September 2012

17. Facadio Antero, M, O'Sullivan, D, Mandavavilli, S, Mullins, J, High prevalence of endometriosis in patients with histologically proven adenomyosis Fertility and Sterility VOLUME 107, ISSUE 3, SUPPLEMENT , E 46, MARCH 01, 201

18. Donnez, J, Donnez, O and Dolmans, M.M., Uterine adenomyosis, another enigmatic disease of our time Fertility and Sterility® Vol. 109, No. 3, March 2018

19. Gordts, S Grimbizis, G and Campo, R. Symptoms and classification of uterine adenomyosis, including the place of hysteroscopy in diagnosis Fertility and Sterility® Vol. 109, No. 3, March 2018

20. Taran, FA,Weaver, A.L.,Coddington, CC and Stewart, E.A. Understanding adenomyosis: a case control study Fertility and Sterilityâ Vol. 94, No. 4, September 2010 Taran, FA,Weaver, A.L.,Coddington, C.C. and Stewart, E.A.

21. Bechtold, E, Naik, AG, Laveaux, SM, Adeleye, a limited differences in the incidence or endometriosis and adenomyosis in black verus white women with pelvic pain. Fertility and Sterility Vol. 116, No. 3, Supplement, September 2021

CHAPTER VIII
Cancer and Endometriosis

1. Hummelshoj,L, Kvaskoff, M, Horne, A Missmer, S., Endometriosis and cancer, endometriosis.org, 2018
2. Králíčková, M, Losan, P, Vetvicka, V,Endometriosis and cancer, Womens Health (2014) 10(6)
3. Simmen, RCM, Quick, CM, Kelley, AS, and Zheng, W Endometriosis and Endometriosis-Associated Tumors, https://www.researchgate.net/publication/July 2019
4. Melin, A, Sparén, P, Persson, I,Bergqvist,A Endometriosis and the risk of cancer with special emphasis on ovarian cancer, Human Reproduction Vol.21, No.5 pp. 1237–1242, 200
5. Anglesio, MS, Papadopoulos, N, Ayhan, A, Cancer-associated mutations in endometriosis without cancer. N Engl J Med. 2017; 376: 1835-1848
6. Pavone ME, Lyttle, B,M, Endometriosis and ovarian cancer: links, risks, and challenges faced, international journal of women's health, 2015:7
7. Kim, HS., Kim, TH., Chung, HH., Song, YS., Risk and prognosis of ovarian cancer in women with endometriosis: a meta-analysis. Br J Cancer. 2014; 110: 1878-1890
8. Kim, HS, Kim, TH, Chung, HH, Song, YS., Risk and prognosis of ovarian cancer in women with endometriosis: a meta-analysis. Br J Cancer. 2014; 110: 1878-1890
9. Ballweg, ML, Overcoming endometriosis, new help from the endometriosis association, Endometriosis Association, Lincolnwood,1987

10. Mostoufizadeh, Mahpareh and Scully, RE, Malignant tumors arising in endometriosis clincal ob and gyn 23; 3 sep. 1980

11.Wang, C, Liang, Z Liu, X, Zhang, Q, Li, S The association between endometriosis, tubal ligation, hysterectomy and epithelial ovarian cancer: meta-analyses.Int J Environ Res Public Health. 2016; 13: E1138

12. Dahiya, A, Endometriosis and malignancy: The intriguing relationship, international journal of gynecology, *International Journal of Gynecology* & *Obstetrics* · Volume 155, Issue 1 2021

13. Mogensen, JB Kjær, SK Mellemkjær, L Jensen, A, Endometriosis and risks for ovarian, endometrial and breast cancers: A nationwide cohort study, Gynecologic Oncology Volume 143, Issue 1, October 2016

14. Hermens, M; van Altena, AM; Velthuis, I; van de Laar,, D.C.M; Bulten, J; van Vliet, Endometrial Cancer Incidence in Endometriosis and Adenomyosis. Cancers 2021, 13, 4592.

15. Brinton LA, Gridley G, Persson I, Baron J, Endometriosis and non-Hodgkin's lymphoma, hospital discharge diagnosis of endometriosis. Am J Obstet Gynecol 1997;176:

16. Farland, LV,Lorrain, S,Missmer, SA, Dartois, L, Endometriosis and the risk of skin cancer: a prospective cohort study, Cancer Causes Control 2017 October, 28(10):1011, 1019

17. National Cancer Institute, SEER cancer statistics review (CSR) 1975–2014. https://seer.cancer.gov/csr/1975_2014, Date: April 2017

18. Brilhante, A,V,M, Lustosa, KA, Cava Portela, MC, Sucupira, LCG, Endometriosis and Ovarian Cancer: an Integrative

Review (Endometriosis and Ovarian Cancer) *Asian Pac J Cancer Prev,* 18 (1),

19. Kvaskoff, M Mu, F, Terry, KL Endometriosis: a high-risk population for major chronic diseases? Hum Reprod Update. 2015; 21: 500-516

CHAPTER IX
Race and Endometriosis

1. Blinick G & Merendino VJ 1951 The infrequency of pelvic endometriosis in Negro women. *American Journal of Surgery* 81 635–636. (https://doi.org/10.1016/0002-9610(51)90153-5)

2. Chatman DL 1976 Endometriosis in the black woman. *American Journal of Obstetrics and Gynecology* 125 987–989. (https://doi.org/10.1016/0002- 9378(76)90502-0)

3. Bougie O, Healey J & Singh SS 2019*a* Behind the times: revisiting endometriosis and race. *American Journal of Obstetrics and Gynecology* 221 35.e1–35.e5. (https://doi.org/10.1016/j.ajog.2019.01.238)

4. Wilson, E 1987 Endometriosis, New York, NY, Alan R. Liss,

5. Hoberman J 2012 Black 7 the Origins and Consequences of Medical Racism. University of California Press.

6. Yearby, R 2020 Structural Racism: The Root Cause of the Social Determinants of Health Structural Racism and Health, Disparities: Reconfiguring the Social Determinants of Health Framework to Include the Root Cause, 48 J. of L. Med. & Ethics 518-526

252 | REFERENCES

7. Gannon R, 2016 Race Is a Social Construct, Scientists Argue, Racial categories are weak proxies for genetic diversity and need to be phased out, LiveScience

8. Dubois, WE, The Health and Physique of the American Negro, University of Massachusetts Amherst Libraries, 1909.

9. W E. B. 1868-1963 Du Bois, The Health and Physique of the Negro American: Report of a Social Study Made Under the Direction of Atlanta University: Atlanta, 1906

10. New AMA policies recognize race as a social, not biological, construct Nov 16 2020 https://www.ama-assn.org/press-center/press-releases/new-ama-policies-recognize-race-social-not-biological-construct

11. Lloyd F, 1964 Endometriosis in the Negro Woman *American Journal of Obstetrics & Gynecology* Volume 89, Issue 4.

12. Kyama MC, D'Hooghe TM, Debrock S, Machoki J, Chai DC, Mwenda JM. 2004 The prevalence of endometriosis among african-american and african-indigenous women. Gynecol Obstet Invest. 57(1):40-2.

13. Chatman DL. 1976 Endometriosis and the black woman. J Reprod. Med.;16(6):303-6.

14. Curlin, J 2020 Racial disparities in endometriosis diagnosis: A conversation, https://blog.flexfits.com/racial-disparities-endometriosis-diagnosis/

15. How race/ethnicity influences endometriosis May 22, 2019 Bob Kronemyer https://www.contemporaryob-gyn.net/view/how-raceethnicity-influences-endometriosis

16. Weed JC 1955 Endometriosis in the Negro. *Annals of Surgery* 141 615–620. (https://doi.org/10.1097/00000658-195505000-00006)

17. Jacoby VL, Fujimoto VY, Giudice LC, Kuppermann M, Washington AE. 2010 Racial and ethnic disparities in benign gynecologic conditions and associated surgeries. Am J Obstet Gynecol. 202(6):514-21.

18. Bougie O, Yap MI, Sikora L, Flaxman T & Singh S 2019*b* Influence of race/ethnicity on prevalence and presentation of endometriosis: a systematic review and meta-analysis. *BJOG* 126 1104–1115. (https:// doi.org/10.1111/1471-0528.15692)

19. Berman, C 2020 Race and Endometriosis: Exploring Myths and Misconceptions Endometriosis Summit https://theendometriosissummit.com/blog/race-and-endometriosisexploring-myths-and-misconceptions/

20. Green, A Carney, D Pallin, D Ngo, L Raymond, K Iezzoni, L and Banaji, M 2007 Implicit Bias among Physicians and its Prediction of Thrombolysis Decisions for Black and White Patients Society of General Internal Medicine;22:1231–1238

21. Williams, D Mohammed, S Leavell, J and Collins, C 2002 Race, socioeconomic status, and health: Complexities, ongoing challenges, and research opportunities Ann. N.Y. Acad. Sci. ISSN 0077-8923

22. Dai Y, Li X, Shi J, Leng J. 2018 A review of the risk factors, genetics and treatment of endometriosis in Chinese women: A comparative update. Reprod Health.21;15(1):82,018-0506 7.

23. Williams, D 2002 Racial/Ethnic Variations in Women's Health: The Social Embeddedness of Health, Vol 92, No. 4 | American Journal of Public Health

24. Bougie, O, Nwosu, I 2022 Revisiting the impact of race/ethnicity in endometriosis Reprod Fertil. 3(2): R34–R41.

254 | REFERENCES

25. Bullard, R Mohai, P Saha, R Wright, B 2007 Toxic Wastes and
   Race at Twenty 1987—2007 A Report Prepared for the
   United Church of Christ Justice & Witness Ministries,
   .United Church of Christ ©
26. Rumph, J Stephens, V Martin, J. Brown, L Thomas, P Cooley, A
   Osteen, K and. Bruner-Tran, K 2022 ,* Uncovering Evi-
   dence: Associations between Environmental Contaminants
   and Disparities in Women's Health *Int. J. Environ. Res.
   Public Health,* 19, 1257

CHAPTER X
Unnecessary Hysterectomies

1. Wright, J, Herzog, T, Tsui, J, Amanth, C, Lewin, S, Nationwide
   Trends in the Performance of Inpatient Hysterectomy in
   the United States, Obstet Gynecol. 2013 Aug; 122(2 0 1):
   233–241. doi: 10.1097/AOG.0b013e318299a6cf
2. Corona, L, Swenson, C, Sheetz, K Campbell, D, DeLancey, J
   Morgan, D, Use of other treatments before hysterectomy
   for benign conditions in a statewide hospital collaborative,
   December
   23,2014DOI:https://doi.org/10.1016/j.ajog.2014.11.031
3. Bower, J, Schreiner, P Sternfeld, B and Lewis, C, Black–White
   Differences in Hysterectomy Prevalence: The CARDIA
   Study, Am J Public Health. 2009 February; 99(2): 300–307.
   doi: 10.2105/AJPH.2008.133702
4. Kjerulff 1,K, Guzinski, G Langenberg, P, Stolley, P, Moye, N Ka-
   zandjian, V, Hysterectomy and race , Obstet Gynecol 1993
   Nov;82(5):757-64.

ENDOMETRIOSIS | 255

5. http://www.doctorsforwomenpllc.com/FromtheDoctorsDesk/tabid/37363/ContentPubID/103792/settmid/79850/Default

6. The American College of Obstetricians and Gynecologists COMMITTEE OPINION Number 701 • June (Reaffirmed 2019) Committee on Gynecologic Practice

7. Clarke-Pearson, D, Geller, E, Complications of hysterectomy, Obstet Gynecol2013 Mar;121(3):654-673.doi: 10.1097/AOG.0b013e3182841594

8. https://www.nhs.uk/conditions/hysterectomy/risks/

9. Danesh, M. Hamzehgardeshi, Z., Moosazadeh, M. and Shabani-Asrami F., The Effect of Hysterectomy on Women's Sexual Function: a Narrative Review, Med Arch. 2015 Dec; 69(6): 387–392.

10. https://hersfoundation.org

11. Schlaff, W, Elagolix for Heavy Menstrual Bleeding in Women with Uterine Fibroids, N Engl J Med 2020;382:328-40.

12. Al-Hendy, A, Lukes, A, Treatment of Uterine Fibroid Symptoms with Relugolix Combination Therapy, N Engl J Med 2021; 384:630-642

13. Taylor, H, Giudice, L, Treatment of Endometriosis-Associated Pain with Elagolix, an Oral GnRH Antagonist, N Engl J Med 2017;377:28-40.

14. https://www.womenshealth.gov/a-z-topics/hysterectomy#3

15 Stringer, N, Uterine Fibroids, What every woman needs to know, Physicians and Scientist Publishing Co, 1996, Glenview, IL

16 Skilling, J, Fibroids, "An Essential Guide for the Newly Diagnosed," Marlowe and Company, 2002, New York, NY

256 | REFERENCES

17. West, S, The Hysterectomy Hoax, Next Decade Pub., Chester, NJ, 2002

CHAPTER XI
How Endometriosis is Diagnosed

1. Broster, A, Why It Takes So Long To Be Diagnosed With Endometriosis, According To An Expert, Aug 27, 2020, HTTPS://WWW.FORBES.COM/SITES/ALICE-BROSTER/2020/08/27/WHY-IT-TAKES-SO-LONG-TO-BE-DIAGNOSED-WITH-ENDOMETRIOSIS-ACCORDING-TO-A-EXPERT/?SH=175F5BB69674

2. Guidice, L, Endometriosis, N Engl J.Med 362;25 nejm.org June 24, 2010

3. https://drseckin.com/symptoms-and-signs-of-endometriosis/

4. *Vercellini P, Trespidi L, De Giorgi O, Cortesi I, Parazzini F, Crosignani PG (1996). "Endometriosis and pelvic pain: relation to disease stage and localization". Fertil Steril. 65 (2): 299–304. PMID 8566252.*

5. *Faley, K,* Quiz: Do I have endometriosis?, April 20, 2022, https://www.osfhealthcare.org/blog/quiz-do-i-have-endometriosis/

6. Mounsey, A, Wilgus, A, Slawson, D, Diagnosis and Management of Endometriosis, Volume 74, Number 4 www.aafp.org/afp American Family Physician, August 15, 2006

7. AGARWAL,SK, CLINICAL DIAGNOSIS OF ENDOMETRIOSIS: A CALL TO ACTION, AM J OB GYN Volume 220, Issue 4, April 2019

8. Wilson, E, Endometriosis, Alan Liss, New York 1987

9. Sutton, C, Modern management of endometriosis, CRC press,Boca Raton, 2011

10. American College of Obstetricians and Gynecologists (ACOG). (2019). *Endometriosis.* https://www.acog.org/Patients/FAQs/Endometriosis ttps://journals.lww.com/green-journal/Citation/2010/07000/Practice_Bulletin_No__114__Management_of.41.aspx

11. Nezhat, C Endometriosis advanced management and surgical techniques, Springer=Verlag, new York 1995

12. Zondervan, K, Becker, C, Missmer, S, Endometriosis, *Nature Reviews Disease Primers* volume 4, Article number: 9 (2018)

13. Garcia-Velasco, J, Endometriosis Current Management and Future Trends, Jaypee Brothers Medical Pub. St. Louis, Mo 2010

14. Waller, K, Shaw, R, Risk Factors for Endometriosis: Menstrual and Life-Style, Med Principles Practice 1998

15. https://www.nichd.nih.gov/health/topics/endometri/condition-info/at-risk

16. Boyles, S, Endometriosis Linked to Other Diseases Fibromyalgia, Chronic Fatigue Common in Women With Endometriosis, https://www.webmd.com/women/endometriosis/news/20020926/endometriosis-linked-to-other-diseases

17. https://www.advancedgynaecologymelbourne.com.au/endometriosis/diagnosis

18. Giudice, L, Endometriosis, Science and Practice, Wiley-Blackwell, West Sussex, UK, 2012

19. Olive, D, Francis, T, Endometriosis Clinical Practice, Med Principles Pract, London 2005

20. Speer, L, CA 125 Relatively Specific for Diagnosing Endometriosis Patient-Oriented Evidence That Matters, Am Fam Physician. 2017;95(2):122

21. Nezhat, C, Endometriosis, Advance Management and Surgical Techniques, springer-Verlag, New York, 1995

22. Zondervan, K, Becker, C, Missmer, S, Endometriosis, n engl j med 382;13 nejm.org, March 26, 2020

CHAPTER XII
How Endometriosis is Treated

1. Gemmell, LC, The management of menopause in women with a history of endometriosis: a systematic review, Human Reproduction Update, Vol.23, No.4 pp. 481–500, 2017

2. Taylor, HS, Treatment of Endometriosis-Associated Pain with Elagolix, an Oral GnRH Antagonist, N Engl j Med 377;1 nejm.org July 6, 2017

3. Acién, Pedro, Endometriosis: A Disease That Remains Enigmatic, Hindawi Publishing Corporation, ISRN Obstetrics and Gynecology, Volume 2013, Article ID 242149

4. Barbieri, RL, Optimize the medical treatment of endometriosis— Use all available medications, OBG Management | August 2018 | Vol. 30 No. 8

5. Taylor, HS New Frontiers in the Management of Endometriosis and Uterine Fibroids: Clinical Highlights from Florence, Medical Learning Institute, Inc. and PVI, PeerView Institute for Medical Education

6. García-Gómez, E Regulation of Inflammation Pathways and Inflammasome by Sex Steroid Hormones in Endometriosis,

Frontiers in Endocrinology | www.frontiersin.org 1 January 2020 | Volume 10 | Article 935

7. Gupta, S, Endometriosis A Comprehensive Update, Springer, New York, 2015

8. https://www.brighamandwomens.org/obgyn/infertility-reproductive-surgery/endometriosis/medical-treatment-for-endometriosis

9. Olive, D, Taylor, F Endometriosis Clinical Practice, London 2005

10. Mangtani, P Epidemiology of endometriosis, Journal of Epidemiology and Community Health 1993; 47: 84-88

11. Luciano, DE, Luciano, A Management of Endometriosis-Related Pain: An Update, Women's Health 2011 Sep;7(5):585-90.

12. The Johns Hopkins Manual of Gynecology and Obstetrics, Lippincott, New York, 2002

13. Davila, W, Endometriosis Treatment & Management Updated: May 10, 2021

14. https://emedicine.medscape.com/article/271899-treatment#d7

15. Taylor, H, Speroff's Clinical Gynecologic Endocrinology and Infertility, Wolters Kluwer 9th edition, Philadelphia 2020

16. Gibson, D, Simitsidellis, I Collins, F and Saunders, P, Endometrial Intracrinology: estrogens, Androgens and Endometrial Disorders, . Int. J. Mol. Sci. 2018, 19, 3276

17. https://www.fiercebiotech.com/biotech/organon-keeps-pedal-to-metal-buying-up-forendo-3rd-deal-since-spinning-out-merck

18. Barbieri, RL, Elagolix: A new treatment for pelvic pain caused by endometriosis, OBG Management | November 2018 | Vol. 30 No. 11

19. ACOB Practice Bulletin no. 114, management of endometriosis, 2010; 223-226

20. Practice Committee of ASRM, treatment of pelvic pain associated with endometriosis; Fert Steril, 2014, 101; 927-935

21. Giudice, LC, Endometriosis: Expert answers to 7 crucial questions on diagnosis, OBG Management | April 2015 | Vol. 27 No. 4

22. Zondervan, K, Endometriosis, N Engl J Med 2020;382:1244-56. DOI: 10.1056/NEJMra1810764

23. Capezzuoli, T, Classification/staging systems for endometriosis: the state of the art, Gynecological and Reproductive Endocrinology and Metabolism 2020; 1(1):14-22

24. https://www.advancedgynaecologymelbourne.com.au/endometriosis/diagnosis

25. https://www.advancedgynaecologymelbourne.com.au/endometriosis/stages

26. Bedaiwy, MA, New developments in the medical treatment of endometriosis, Fertility and Sterility® Vol. 107, No. 3, March 2017 0015-0282/$36.00

27. Ezzat, L, Medical treatment of endometriosis: an update, *Int J Reprod Contracept Obstet Gynecol. 2017 Oct;6(10):4187-4192*

CHAPTER XIII
Alternative Ways to Repress Endometriosis

1. Taylor, HS, Giudice, L C, Lessey, BA, Abrao, MS, Treatment of Endometriosis-Associated Pain with Elagolix, an Oral GnRH Antagonist, N Engl J Med 2017;377:28-40.

2. Zondervan, K, Becker, C, Missmer, S Endometriosis N Engl J Med 2020;382:1244-56.
3. Cook, A, Stop Endometriosis and Pelvic Pain, Femsana Press, Los Gatos, CA 2012
4. https://www.brighamandwomens.org/obgyn/infertility-reproductive-surgery/endometriosis/complimentary-and-alternative-therapies-for-endometriosis
5. Guo, Y, Liu, F-Y, Complementary and Alternative Medicine for Dysmenorrhea Caused by Endometriosis: A Review of Utilization and Mechanism
6. Kong, S, Zhang, Y The Complementary and Alternative Medicine for Endometriosis: A Review of Utilization and Mechanism
7. Paiva S, Carneiro, MM Complementary and Alternative Medicine in the Treatment of Chronic Pelvic Pain in Women: What Is the Evidence? ISRN Pain. 2013; 2013:469575. Published 2013 Nov 28. doi:10.1155/2013/469575.
8. Kold M, Hansen T, Vedsted-Hansen H, Forman A Mindfulness-based psychological intervention for coping with pain in endometriosis. Nordic Psychology. 2012; 64(1), 2-16.
9. Gonçalves AV, Makuch MY, Setubal MS, Barros NF, Bahamondes L. A Qualitative Study on the Practice of Yoga for Women with Pain-Associated Endometriosis. J Altern Complement Med. 2016;22(12):977-982. doi:10.1089/acm.2016.0021.
10. Ghonemy, G and Sharkawy, N, Impact of Changing Lifestyle on Endometriosis Related Pain, Journal of Nursing and Health Science (IOSR-JNHS e-ISSN: 2320–1959.p- ISSN: 2320–1940 Volume 6, Issue 2 Ver. V (Mar. - Apr. 2017),

262 | REFERENCES

11. Signorello, L,

12. Nirgianakis, K Egger, K, Effectiveness of Dietary Interventions in the Treatment of Endometriosis: a Systematic Review, Reproductive Sciences (2022) 29:26–42

13. The Best and Worst Foods for an Anti-Inflammatory Endometriosis,https://health.clevelandclinic.org/endometriosis-diet/

14. Is there a universal diet for Endometriosis? https://www.endometriosisaustralia.org/post/is-there-a-universal-diet-for-endometriosis

15. Karlsson, V, Experiences of health after dietary changes in endometriosis: a qualitative interview study, BMJ Open 2020;10:e032321. doi:10.1136/bmjopen-2019-032321

16. Foods That Can Help Endometriosis (and 6 to Avoid) https://greatist.com/eat/endometriosis-diet-tips#bottom-line

17. Endometriosis Diet Tips That May Help You Manage Symptoms, According to Expertshttps://www.health.com/condition/endometriosis/endometriosis-diet

18. https://avivaromm.com/endometriosis-herbs-supplements/

19. Ratini, M, Herbs for Endometriosis, June 16, 2021, https://www.webmd.com/women/endometriosis/herbs-for-endometriosis

20 Mohd, DA, Kamal Salamt, N, Beneficial Effects of Green Tea Catechins on Female Reproductive Disorders: A Review, Molecules Volume 26 Issue 9 10.3390/molecules26092675

21.Man, G Hui Xu and Wang, C, Green Tea for Endometriosis, Endometriosis - Basic Concepts and Current Research

Trends, http://www.intechopen.com/books/endometriosis-basic-concepts-and-current-research- trends/green-tea-for-endometriosis

22. Dull, A Moga, A, Therapeutic Approaches of Resveratrol on Endometriosis via Anti-Inflammatory and Anti-Angiogenic Pathways, *Molecules* 2019, *24*, 667; doi:10.3390/molecules24040667

23. https://www.endonews.com/resveratrol-and-endometriosis-Bottom of Form Bottom of Form

24. Halpern, G, Chor, E Kopelman, A, Nutritional aspects related to endometriosis, rev asso C Med Bras 2015; 61(6):519-523

CHAPTER XIV
Adolescents and Endometriosis

1. Endometriosis Association, https://endometriosisassn.org/endometriosis-resources/teens

2. Balun, J, Dominick, K, Cabral, MD, Taubel, T, Endometriosis in adolescents, Pediatr Med 2019;2:33

3. Hull, L, Adolescent Endometriosis, Endometriosis Australia's Clinical Advisory Member 2017 #1in10 #endoblog #endometriosisawareness #endoawareness #pelvicpain #endometriosisblog #womenshealth #endoaustralia #endofacts #endometriosis #endo

4. Dun, E C, Kho, KA, Morozov, VV, Kearney, S, Zurawin, JL, Nezhat, CH, Endometriosis in Adolescents: Referrals, Diagnosis, Treatment, and Outcomes, April-June 2015 Volume 19 Issue 2 e2015.00019 1 JSLS www.SLS.org

264 | REFERENCES

5. Cook, AS, stop Endometriosis and pelvic pain, Femsana Press Los Gatos, CA, 2012

6. Wilson, EA, Endometriosis, Alan R. Liss, New York, 1987

7. ACOG dysmenorrhea and endometriosis in the adolescent ACOG committee on adolescent health no. 760, December vol 132, no 6, December 2018

8. Dessole, M, Melis, GB, Angioni S, Endometriosis in Adolescence Obstet Gynecol Int. 2012; 2012: 869191. Published online 2012 Oct 10. doi: 10.1155/2012/869191

9. Sachedina, A, Todd, N, Dysmenorrhea, Endometriosis and Chronic Pelvic Pain in Adolescents J Clin Res Pediatr Endocrinol. 2020 Jan; 12(Suppl 1): 7–17. Published online 2020 Feb 6. doi: 10.4274/jcrpe.galenos.2019.2019.S0217

10. Seckin, T, Recognizing and Treating Endometriosis, Turner publishing co, Nashville, TN 2016

11. Ballweg, ML, Endometriosis The complete reference for taking charge of your health, contemporary books, 2004

12. Krotec, J, Endometriosis for Dummies, Wiley Pub, 2007

13. Agarwal, SK, Chapron, C, Clinical diagnosis of endometriosis: a call to action, American Journal of Ob & Gyn, April 2019

14. Zondervan, KT, Becker, CM, Missmer, SA, Endometriosis, N Engl J Med 382;13 nejm.org March 26, 2020

15. Garcia-Velasco, JA, Rizk, BRMB, Endometriosis current management and future trends, Jaypee Brothers St. Louis, 2010

16. Giudice, LC, Evers, JLH., Healy, DL, Endometriosis, science and practice, Wiley-Blackwell, West Sussex, UK, 2012

17. Nezhat, CH, Endometriosis in Adolescents, Springer, Cham Switzerland, 2020

CHAPTER XV
Distant Endometriosis

1. Jubanyik, KJ, Comite, F, Extrapelvic Endometriosis, Obstetrics an Gynecology Clinics of North America, Vol. 24, Issue 2, June 1997

2. Machairiotis, N, Stylianaki, A, Dryllis, G, Zarogoulidis, P, Extrapelvic Endometriosis, a rare entity or an under diagnosed condition? Diagnostic Pathology, Dec. 2013

3. Charatsi, D, Koukoura, O, Ntavela, I G, Chintziou, F, Gastrointestinal and Urinary Tract Endometriosis: A Review on the Commonest Locations of Extrapelvic Endometriosis, Adv. Med. Sep. 2018

4. Chan, DL, Chua, D, Ravindran, P, Cerdeira, MP, Mor, I, A case report of endometriosis presenting as an acute small bowel obstruction, Int. J. Surg Case Rep. Oct. 2017;41

5. Iwakawa, k, Nonoshita, T, Hamada, Y, Yasui, N, A Report of Four Cases of Intestinal Endometriosis, Hiroshima Journal of Medical, Vol. 66, Issue 2, 2017

6. Fadil, A, Case report and video presentation: Trans-urethral resection of bladder endometriosis Urology Case Reports, vol. 24, May 2019

7. Leonardi, M, Espada, M, Kho, RM, Magrina, JF, Millischer, A, E, Endometriosis and the Urinary Tract: From Diagnosis to Surgical Treatment, Diagnostics (Basel). Oct. 2020 Oct;

8. Sutton, C, Modern Management of Endometriosis, CR Press, Boca Raton, 2019

9. Bridge-Cook, P Thoracic Endometriosis, https://www.hormonesmatter.com/support-hormones-matter/ April 2, 2018

266 | REFERENCES

10. Nezhat, C, Hajhosseini, B,Buescher, E, Hussein, A, Hilaris, GE, Sellin, M,Thoracic Endometriosis Syndrome Prevention and Management, JSLS Journal October 2018

11. Azizad-Pinto, P, Clarke, D, Thoracic Endometriosis Syndrome: Case Report and Review of the Literature, Perm J 2014 Summer;18

12. Hirata, T, Koga, K, Osuga, Y, Extra-pelvic endometriosis: A review Reprod Med Biol.2020;19:

13. Chamie, LP, Ferreira, DM, Ribeiro, R, Fiferes, DA, Atypical Sites of Deeply Infiltrative Endometriosis: Clinical Characteristics and Imaging Findings[1]RadioGraphics 2018;

14. Bennett, GL, Slywotzky, CM, Cantera, M, Hecht, EM, Unusual Manifestations and Complications of Endometriosis— Spectrum of Imaging Findings: *Pictorial Review* AJR:194, June 2010

CHAPTER XVI
Clinical Trials

1. https://www.nih.gov/health-information/nih-clinical-research-trials-you/basics

2. https://www.ed.ac.uk/centre-reproductive-health/exppect-endometriosis/welcome/why-participate-in-trials-for-endometriosis 24 august 2020

3. East C, Developing a Successful Clinical Research Program, Springer, Cham, Switzerland 2018

4. Depoy, E, Gitlin, LN, Introduction to Research, Understanding and Applying multiple Strategies, Elsevier Mosby, St. Louis, MO, 2005

ENDOMETRIOSIS | 267

5. https://www.nia.nih.gov/health/what-are-clinical-trials-and-studies
6. https://www.fda.gov/patients/drug-development-process/step-3-clinical-research
7. Horne AW, et al. Top ten research priorities in the UK and Ireland. Lancet 2017;389:2191-92
8. Malvezzi, H, Marengo, EB, Podgaec , S, Piccinato, C, Endometriosis: current challenges in modeling a multifactorial disease of unknown etiology *Journal of Translational Medicine* volume 18, Article number: 311 (2020)

CHAPTER XVII
Case Histories

CHAPTER XVIII
Endometriosis Awareness

1. Kronfeld, H, How Did Endo Awareness Month Begin? Five Fast Facts, March 7, 2018 https://www.endofound.org/how-did-endo-awareness-month-begin-five-fast-facts
2. Ellis K, Munro D, Clarke J, Endometriosis Is Undervalued: A Call to Action, Frontiers in Global Women's Health May 2022 | Volume 3
3. She Has Given the World Three Great Gifts: Mary Lou Ballweg Our Bodies Our Selves https://www.ourbodiesourselves.org/blog/she-has-given-the-world three-great-gifts-mary-lou-ballweg/ May 2, 2009
4. https://endometriosisassn.org/profile/mary-lou-ballweg
5. https://www.webmd.com/mary-lou-ballweg

268 | REFERENCES

6. Ballweg, ML, Impact of endometriosis on women's health: comparative historical data show that the earlier the onset, the more severe the disease, ePract Res Clin Obstet Gynaecol Apr 2004

CHAPTER XIX
The Future

1. Ellis K, Munro D, Clarke J, Endometriosis Is Undervalued: A Call to Action, Frontiers in Global Women's Health May 2022 | Volume 3
2. Thomas, E, Rock, J, Modern Approaches to Endometriosis, Springer Science, 2003
3. Horne, A, Saunders, PTK, Abokjhrais, IM, Hogg, L, Top ten endometriosis research priorities in the UK and Ireland, www.thelancet.com, May 19, 2017
4. Oransay, S, Endometriosis Prediction by Machine Learning, Journal of Personalized Medicine, September 30, 2022
5. Blass, I.; Sahar, T.; Shraibman, A.; Ofer, D.; Rappoport, N.; Linial, M. Revisiting the Risk Factors for Endometriosis: A Machine Learning Approach. J. Pers. Med. 2022, 12, 1114. https://doi.org/ 10.3390/jpm12071114
6. Bendifallah, S, Dabil, Y, Suisse,S, Jornea, L MicroRNome analysis generates a blood-based signature for endometriosis, Scientific Reports | (2022)
7. Dabi, Y.; Suisse, S.;Jornea, L., Bouteiller, D.; Touboul, C.; Puchar, A.; Daraï, E.; Bendifallah, S. Clues for Improving the Pathophysiology Knowledge for Endometriosis Using Serum Micro-RNA Expression. *Diagnostics* 2022,12,175. https://doi.org/ 10.3390/diagnostics12010175

8. Guerriero, S, Pascual, M, Ajossa, S, Graupera, B, Artificial intelligence in the detection of endometriosis of uterosacral ligaments

9. Iftikhar P M, Kuijpers M V, Khayyat A, et al. (February 28, 2020) Artificial Intelligence: A New Paradigm in Obstetrics and Gynecology Research and Clinical Practice. Cureus 12(2): e7124. DOI 10.7759/cureus.7124

10. Nouri, B, Roshandel, S Is Artificial Intelligence a New Diagnostic Approach for Patients with Endometriosis? Interv Pain Med Neuromod. August 10, 2022

11. Berthelot, S, MIT event illuminate critical need for menstruation science, Center for Gynepathology Research, October 3, 2022

12. Moawad, G, Exploring the potential of AI for gynecologic surgery, AAGL November 15, 2021

13. Sivajohan, B, Elgendi, M, Menon, C, Allaire, C, Clinical use of artificial intelligence in endometriosis: a scoping review, npj Digital Medicine (2022) 5:109   www.nature.com/npjdigitalmed

14. Avery, J, Imagendo; AI to improve endometriosis diagnosis, 2020 https://imagendo.org.au/

15. Haug, CJ, Drazen, JM, Artificial intelligence and Machine Learning in Clinical Medicine, 2023, NEJM 2023;388;1201-8

16. Beam, AL, Drazen, JM, Kohane, IS, Leong, TY, Artificial Intelligence in Medicine, NEJM, March 30, 2023

17. Lee, P, Bubeck, S., Petro, J, Benefits, Limits and Risks of GPT-4 as an AI Chatbot for medicine, NEJM, March 30, 2023

18. Haupt, CE, Mason, M, AI-Generated Medical Advice—GPT and Beyond, JAMA, March 27, 2023

Index

Abdominal, 88
    hysterectomy, 88, 89, 90
    or laparotomy
myomectomy, 58
Abnormal, 43
    fertilization and
    implantation, 43
    utero-tubal transport, 43
Acupuncture, 122
Adenomyoma, 7
Adenomyomectomy, 66
Adenomyosis, 61, 62, 87
    diagnosing, 63
    medication for, 64
    surgery for, 65
    treatment of, 64, 65
Adhesions, 6
African American women, 81
Air pollution, 30
Alcohol, 128
Alterations to the
microbiome, 179
Altered Systemic Immune
Function, 42
Aluminum, 27
American Journal of
Epidemiology, 22
American Medical Association
(AMA), 80
American Society for
Reproductive Medicine
(ASRM), 107, 117
    endometriosis stages, 118

Apoptosis, 15
    suppression, 17
Aromatase Inhibitors, 114,
Arsenic, 27
Artificial intelligence (AI), 179,
180
Asian women, 81, 82
Augmented reality, 179, 180
Beauty product exposures, 23
Biofeedback, 123
Black women, 21, 22, 81, 82
Bottled water, 26,
Breast cancer, 74, 76
Caffeine, 128
Cancer Alley, 20
Cancer Antigen-125 (CA 125),
105
Cancer, 76, 88
    reducing risks of, 76
Carbon dioxide (C02) laser, 57
Carl von Rokitansky, 7
Chocolate cysts, 6, 17
Cleaning products, 29
Clinical study, 155
Clinical trials, 151, 152, 153,
154, 155, 158, 159, 160
    benefits of participating in
    a, 160
    concerns and questions,
    153
    how safe are, 160
    importance of, 151
    phases of, 153
    reasons for conducting, 152

Combination therapy, 150
Continuous progestin
hormonal therapy, 112
Cryomyolysis, 57
CT scanning, 105
Curcumin, 129
Danazol, 113
Dartmouth Medical School, 172
Dilation and curettage (D&C), 94
Dioxin, 13, 14, 28
Donald Chatman, 80
Electroacupuncture, 122
Encyclopedia of Ecology, 27
Endocrine and Ovulatory
Abnormalities, 42
Endometrial, 65
    ablation, 65
    cancer, 74
Endometriomas, 6
Endometriosis Awareness
Month (EAM), 172
Endometriosis Priority Setting
Partnership (PSP), 176
Endometriosis, 3, 4, 5, 39, 46, 61, 62, 70, 83, 87, 99, 100, 103, 117, 126, 135, 150, 160, 175
    adenomyosis and, 61, 67
    alternative ways to repress, 121
    and adenomyosis, 7, 166
    and associated cancers, 70
    and endometrial carcinoma, 74
    and fibroids, 163
    and infertility, 167
    and ovarian cyst, 168
    and polycystic ovaries, 164
    and post hysterectomy pain, 165
    and post-menopausal pain, 167
    and uterine fibroids, 50
    associated ovarian cancer, 71, 72
    association, 3, 171
    autoimmune diseases associated with, 38
    awareness, 171
    breast cancer, 74
    cancer and, 69
        symptoms and location, 62
    cancer in women with, 76
    cause of, 11, 12, 17, 31
        apoptosis, 15
        cells, 16
        environmental, 13
        genetics, 12
        hormones, 14, 16
        immune cause of, system, 15
        lymphatic system, 15
        metaplasia, 14, 16
        mulleriosis and embryonic origin theory, 12
        oxidative stress, 15, 16
        Sampson's theory of retrograde menstruation, 12
        stem cell theory, 11
        uterine peristalsis, 14
    clinical diagnosis of, 101
        imaging, 104
        laparoscopy, 106, 107
        medical history, 102

physical examination, 103

serum markers, 105

clinical trials for, 184

common locations of, 144

common symptoms, 50, 52, 61, 62, 70

conventional diagnosis of, 106

definition, 5

description, 6

diagnosis, 138

distant or extra-pelvic, 143

environmental toxins and, 19

fibroid tumors and, 49, 51

foods that help with, 127

foods to avoid with, 128

history, 7

infertility and, 41

infertility, 36

intestinal, 144

lesions, 6

management, 139

medical management for, 45

medical research, 160

medical treatment of, 44

other cancers and, 75

pain, 35

peritoneal, 17

race and, 79, 99, 100, 103, 117

reduced diagnosis of, 161

risk factors associated with, 137

risk factors for, 103

surgery for the treatment of, 117

surgical management of, 44

symptoms, 4, 35, 37, 38, 39, 137, 138, 183

syndrome, 150

thoracic, 146

top ten research priorities for, 177, 178

treatment of, 109, 148

urinary tract, 145

women with, 78

Environment, 19

role of the, 31

Environmental exposure, 24

mitigation of, 24

Environmental Health, 25

Environmental Protection Agency (EPA), 14, 25

Environmental, 13

Epigallocatechin gallate (EGCG), 132

Epigenetic modifications, 13

Estrogen and progesterone, 14

Estrogen-progestin contraceptives, 111

Exercise and physical activities, 125

Exercises, 92

Exploratory laparotomy, 8

Fatty meat, 128

Fiber, 127

Fibroid tumors, 49, 51

types, 52

Filtered water, 27

Fistula formation, 89

Food and Drug Agency (FDA), 25, 157, 156

Frank Lloyd, 80

Free radicals, 15

Future therapeutics, 114

Genetics, 12

Ginger, 131Gonadotropin-releasing hormone (GnRH)

antagonist, 55, 64, 93, 113, 140, 149

Gonadotropin-releasing hormone agonist (GnRH), 55, 64, 93, 112, 140, 149

Gonadotropin-Releasing Hormone Analogues, 112

Green tea, 132

Gynecologists, 77

Heavy vaginal bleeding, 87

Henry Clarke, 8

HEPA filters, 30, 31

Herbs and supplements, 128

HERS Foundation (Hysterectomy Resources and Educational Services Foundation), 92

High Intensity Focused Ultrasound (HIFU), 65

Hispanic women, 81

Hormonal treatment, 44

Hormones, 14, 16

House plants, 27

Hyperestrogenemia, 71

Hypnosis, 124, 125

Hysterectomy, 58, 66, 85
    abdominal, 88, 89, 90
    adverse effects, 90
    alternatives to, 91
    complications and side effects, 89
    indications for, 86
        adenomyosis, 87
        endometriosis, 87
        heavy vaginal bleeding, 87
        uterine fibroids, 87
        uterine prolapse, 87
    laparoscopic, 88

robotic surgery, 88
    treatment options, 92
    types of, 88
    vaginal, 88

Hysteroscopic myomectomy, 57

Hysteroscopy, 54

Imaging, 104, 139

Immune dysfunction, 17

Immune system, 15

Impaired implantation, 43

Inflammation, 127

Institutional Review Boards (IRB), 156, 157

Killer cramps, 136

Kurt Semm, 8

Laparoscopic, 88
    and laparotomy, 66
    hysterectomy, 88
    or robotic myomectomy, 57
    surgery, 94

Laparoscopy, 8, 9, 45, 106, 107, 117, 140
    diagnostic, 106
    operative, 140
    robotic, 106

Lifestyle modification, 125

Lymphatic system, 15, 17

Machine learning, 179, 180

Magnetic resonance (MR)-guided focused ultrasound (MR[f]US), 95

Magnetic resonance imaging (MRI), 54, 63, 105

Management of infertility, 43

Mary Lou Ballweg, 171, 172, 173

Medical history, 102

Medical treatment, 110, 149

Medical-surgical therapy, 45
Medication, 92
Meditation, 124
Melanoma, 75, 76
Melatonin, 130
Menopausal symptoms, 90
Metaplasia, 14, 16
Mindfulness, 124
Mossville, 21
Moxibustion, 122
Mucosal invasion, 7
Mullerian duct system, 12
Mulleriosis and Embryonic Origin Theory, 12
Myolysis, 95
Myomectomy, 94
N-acetyl-cysteine (NAC), 131, 132
Nanomedicines, 179
National Institute of Health (NIH), 151, 175
New biomarker analysis, 179
Non-Hodgkin's Lymphoma, 75, 76
Nonsteroidal anti-inflammatory medications (NSAIDs), 111
Nutrition, 126
Obstructive reproductive tract abnormalities (Mullerian anomalies), 137
Office of Human Subjects Research Protection, 157
Ovarian cancer, 70, 71, 72, 73, 76
Ovarian endometriosis, 71
Oxidative stress, 15, 16, 131
Pelvic, 42
    adhesions, 42

    anatomy, 42
Pelvic pain, 102
    and infertility, 102
    hormone medication options to treat, 115
Peritoneal function, 42
Physical examination, 103, 139
Physical therapy and massage, 123
Polyethylene terephthalate (PET), 26
Postoperative medical therapy, 45
Preoperative therapy, 45
Probe Directed Pelvic Pain Assessment (PDPPA), 104
Processed foods, 128
Progestins, 111
Pycnogenol (Maritime Pine Bark), 129
Qigong, 124
Radiofrequency ablation, 57
Reproductive Development, 22
Research Priorities, 176
Research Protection, 157
Resveratrol, 133
Retrograde flow, 12
Retrograde menstruation, 16
Reverse osmosis, 27
Robotic surgery, 88
Sampson's Theory of Retrograde Menstruation, 12
Science, 25
Serum markers, 105
Severe painful periods, 136
Sonohysterography, 54
Stem cell theory, 11, 17
Sugary drinks, 128
Surgery, 93, 94

Surgical treatment, 44, 45, 115
Tai Chi, 123, 124
The Endometriosis Awareness Week, 172
The Mossville story, 20
The principle of see and treat, 106
The protocol, 155
The revised ASRM (rASRM) classification system, 117
The Yellow Ribbon, 172
Theory of mulleriosis, 12
Thomas Stephen Cullen, 7, 8
Transcutaneous Electrical Nerve (TEN), 123
Transvaginal ultrasound, 63
Ultrasonography, 104
Ultrasound, 54
USDA organic, 24, 25
Uterine artery embolization (UAE), 56, 65, 95
Uterine fibroids, 22, 50, 53, 87, 92
  diagnosis of, 53
  medications for, 55
  surgery for, 56
    abdominal or laparotomy
  myomectomy, 58
    hysterectomy, 58
    hysteroscopic myomectomy, 57
    laparoscopic or robotic
  myomectomy, 57
    radiofrequency ablation, 57
    Uterine Artery Embolization (UAE), 56
  surgical treatment of, 59

treatment, 55
Uterine, 8
  mucosa, 8
  prolapse, 87
  peristalsis, 14, 17
Vaginal, 88
  hysterectomy, 88
  pessary, 93
Vanderbilt University School of Medicine, 172
Vitamin B6, 133
W.E.B. Du Bois, 79
Water filters, 27
White women, 21, 22, 81, 82
Women's hair products, 21
World Bank's population estimate 2017, 5
Yoga, 123, 124
Yttrium Aluminum Garnet (YAG) laser, 57

Made in the USA
Middletown, DE
21 July 2024